THE MAGIC MUSSEL

— ARTHRITIS ANOTHER WAY

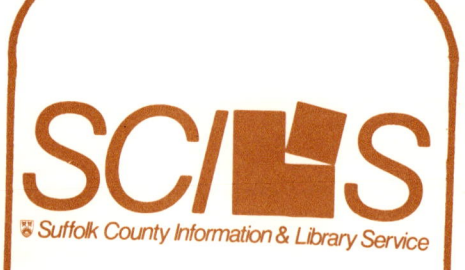

SC/LS
Suffolk County Information & Library Service

THE MAGIC MUSSEL

— ARTHRITIS ANOTHER WAY

BY

DESMOND ZWAR

IDEAS UNLIMITED
CAIRNS, AUSTRALIA. 1983

Copyright © 1983 by Desmond Zwar
All rights reserved, including the right to reproduce this
book or portions thereof in any form.
First published 1983 by Ideas Unlimited, Cairns, Australia.

ISBN 0 946714 01 0

Typeset by Cairns Foto Type, Cairns, Nth. Queensland.

Printed at Griffin Press Limited, Marion Road, Netley, South Australia

FOREWORD

"A new drug went on the market this week that will allow America's 25 million arthritis sufferers to put away their aspirin bottles and find new pain relief with fewer side-effects."

— Newspaper item from New York.

"An arthritis drug which some doctors described as a revolutionary treatment for arthritis has been found to have killed people who have consumed it. It has been withdrawn from sale."

— Television item.

"The number of aching joints in this world is exceeded only by the amount of money which quacks make by pretending to ease them."

— A medical expert on rheumatic diseases.

* * *

Many hands holding newspapers carrying the first message would have resembled claws, with fingers bent permanently inwards from the effects of rheumatoid arthritis. Buttocks belonging to people watching the second item on television would be aching, their owners slumped awkwardly in armchairs, hips and joints throbbing, eyes ringed from lack of sleep or the effects of hypnotic drugs.

"A cure...? That's what they said last time."

My mother has arthritis. Until recently she could move only slowly and painfully a step at a time, leaning heavily on a walking aid. When the phone rang it took her two minutes to get out of her chair. She is 77 and had to be helped to dress and was dependent on others for meals.

She is probably not much worse off than two million other Australians who have had one of the many forms of arthritis, or the millions of Britons and Americans. I mention her only because as her son, and as a writer whose role is investigative reporting, I have a dual responsibility : I must not give false hope. And yet I must not leave information untapped which could one day lead to the alleviation of the pain that she and millions of others suffer. Such investigation by a lay writer is often frustrated by inflexible medical specialists who will not budge from 'established' opinion.

There is, I have found, a yawning chasm between these attitudes and others who will explore avenues that may appear unorthodox. It is a deep valley and is filled often with bitterness and acrimony.

A capsule of New Zealand green-lipped mussel extract, which was slightly odorous despite its enclosure in gelatin, came into my life in 1975. I was lunching with a friend of 30 years and he told me his brother had become involved in helping people suffering from arthritis.

I had known Jim Broadbent as a serious, slightly sardonic businessman whose interests involved motels and supermarkets. But what could he possibly know about *medicine*?

"He's working with a family in Auckland who are breeding green-lipped mussels," said Bill Broadbent. "They're giving them to people with arthritis and they're getting quite astonishing results."

"When the doctors have had a look at it and say it works, let me know," I said.

"I will," promised Bill.

He did. And this book is the result.

CHAPTER ONE

ARTHRITIS — THE DISEASE

Arthritis is a general term, and it covers any inflammation of a joint. There are many different types of arthritis. Doctors know the specific causes of some, but in most cases the reason the disease has appeared is not known. The most common of the 'arthritis' diseases are rheumatoid arthritis and osteoarthritis.

Rheumatoid arthritis is a chronic condition that is usually progressive in nature. It involves inflammation of the joints and may begin suddenly, with inflammation in several joints, or it may be gradual, affecting first one joint and then another. The joints become sore and tender to the touch and are stiff after periods of rest or inactivity; they often become misshapen and swollen.

Osteoarthritis is a degenerating disease of the joints which results in fissures or cracks in articular (joint) cartilage, the glistening, smooth material that lines the bones. It is a 'wear and tear' process and it can occur as a late change following and 'insult' to the joint — including fracture, dislocation or arthritis, including rheumatoid arthritis. It can be a crippling disease if it is severe enough, particularly in the hip, or in the knees or feet. Obesity predisposes to and exacerbates osteoarthritis in weight-bearing joints. A patient with chronic rheumatoid arthritis, which is comparatively long-standing, may have problems due to his inflammatory symptoms, and secondary degenerative joint disease — osteoarthritis — which has developed because of the damage to the joint surface caused by his rheumatoid arthritis. (Medical experts choose to call the disease osteoarthrosis, because 'arthritis' means inflammation of a joint; in 'osteoarthritis', as it is loosely termed, this inflammation can be slight.) Surgery may be required in osteoarthrosis to relieve the crippling effects if there is sufficient disability.

Why do we get rheumatoid arthritis?

Some research scientists believe it is the body actually

fighting itself — an 'auto-immune' disease. Our immune systems can be likened to a police force on duty 24 hours a day. When criminals — like bacteria — break in, our immune system hurriedly despatches 'constables' to get rid of them. But in the arthritic's body something has gone wrong with this usually efficient organisation; the police are confused and go about attacking perfectly innocent citizens: the body's own cells. This angry assault is centred on the joints and causes chronic inflammation. Even though such an attack may be most *apparent* in the joints, the disease affects other organs as well, including connective tissue. This explains why the patient feels so sick. "He has a general disease," says a leading rheumatologist, "not just a disease that affects the joints."

Doctors generally diagnose rheumatoid arthritis on clinical grounds; there may be no changes detectable by x-ray in the early stages of the disease. X-rays and blood tests may contribute later to making a firm diagnosis and can be important in differentiating the forms of arthritis which resemble rheumatoid arthritis. 'ESR' — a blood test which shows the sedimentation rate — is used to follow the progress of rheumatoid arthritis once it has been diagnosed.

Having identified a patient's rheumatoid arthritis, what can the doctor do about helping him? He will, at the moment, have to explain that he can offer no cure, but that he can help control it. About 70 percent of patients improve with either medical or surgical treatment. Others have a less optimistic outlook and some will become incapacitated.

Apart from advising rest, physiotherapy and sometimes splinting, doctors offer anti-inflammatory drugs that reduce the inflammation, swelling and pain. Aspirin is the simplest and often the most effective of these drugs. The aim of the physician is to achieve a certain level of aspirin in the blood that will keep the pain and swelling under control.

Sometimes gold salts, penicillamine and chloroquine are prescribed. They are not anti-inflammatory drugs but can — and often do — cause a remission in rheumatoid arthritis; they have no direct anti-inflammatory effect. Their role is entirely different in action and purpose than the anti-inflammatories. They do not directly relieve pain and stiffness, but they can establish long-term control of the disease by affecting, in some way, the disease process rather than the symptoms of the disease process. If gold salts and penicillamine are used, doctors must perform regular blood and urine tests to watch for side-effects.

Cortisone does not influence the course of the disease and should be used in rheumatoid arthritis only in special circumstances, and only in a minimum dose to make life bearable. It should never be used alone. Unfortunately, the initial dramatic effect of the drug does not persist, and side-effects are inevitable if cortisone is taken in sufficiently high doses for long enough. One side-effect is a 'moon face'; but more seriously it can result in crush fractures due to the softening of the bones, susceptibility to infection (because it suppresses normal immune reactions), exacerbation of diabetes and peptic ulcers, cataracts and fragile skin that bruises easily.

A constant search goes on in laboratories and drug houses around the world for an alternative to drugs with side-effects: a 'magic bullet' that will get to the source of the problem treating not just the results of the arthritic disease, but the *cause*.

In Glasgow, Scotland, in the early 1970's, an 83-year-old woman suffering from rheumatoid arthritis, received in the mail from her friend in New Zealand, a bottle of capsules that had a fishy smell about them. She took them with her when she went to see the physician who had been treating her — without sucess — using conventional and homoeopathic remedies.

It became the first meeting between a doctor with an innovative medical outlook and *Perna canaliculus,* the New Zealand green-lipped mussel.

And it was the beginning of a medical controversy that was to spread across the world.

CHAPTER TWO

FARMING THE MUSSEL

Stuart McFarlane, 47, is a short, lean man with stocky and powerful legs. He has been a fisherman for most of his life, but spent seven years working on the Auckland docks. There he learned to watch his back from attack and steel himself against angry insults from fellow workers whose union had been de-registered.

He had left school at fifteen-and-a-half to join his father, Allan, and his elder brother, Athol, at sea. They fished for the succulent hapuka and swordfish. But it was a hard living and when there was a major dock strike and the promise of work the whole family decided to leave the sea. To get his application approved, Stuart had to put his age up by a year.

It was heavy, monotonous work. Frozen lamb carcasses and crates of butter had to be physically juggled on to slings and into ships' holds. "It got very nasty at times," Stuart recalls. "Whole families were broken up by de-registration of the Union, with father taking sides against son in the dispute. One brother hit another across the face with a chain and blinded him."

At weekends the McFarlanes took to the sea again, fishing from the *"Shenandoah"*, a boat they were still paying for, and hardly adequate to earn them the repayments, let alone a living.

Athol and Stuart badly wanted to get completely away from the wharves but the financial difficulties of relying on fishing for an income were formidable. It was to be four and a-half years before they could quit the docks and return to full-time commercial fishing. Even then McFarlane Snr. stayed on as a wharf-labourer while his sons fished all week on the *"Shenandoah"*, using it at weekends to take amateur fishermen on fishing trips.

One lesson Stuart learned from the weekend work was to avoid alcohol. "I had to clean up after them when they had been drinking in rough weather and it was enough to put me off drink." By now the McFarlanes were concentrating on dredging for the big New Zealand green-lipped mussel, a shellfish measuring up to nine inches long, filled with thick, delicate meat savoured by the Maoris. Auckland fish shops would take all the mussels fishermen could dredge, knowing the Maori demand was enthusiastic and constant; restaurants also had them on their menus. The problem was that mussels were becoming harder to find on the ocean floor. New Zealand waters were being fished out of the molluscs and the *"Shenandoah"* was constantly searching for new commercial grounds. Because it was 55 feet long it was capable of dragging an 11-feet wide dredge which detached and brought up large hauls from the bottom. There were four other main rival boats each about 40-ft. long, and the presence of the McFarlane boat was often resented. There were several blatant attempts to ram the *"Shenandoah"*, and the reaction from Stuart McFarlane was shrewd. "We didn't bother about going to the police. I just took photographs of the other trawlers moving across our bows and took them to the insurance company that insured both of us. They were horrified at the prospect of a double pay-out and the intimidation stopped."

Mussels lie in clumps on the stony bed of the sea and a dredge can bring up more stones than mussels in a lift. With the *"Shenandoah's"* winches hauling up the catch a foot or so at a time, the McFarlanes had to balance on the huge metal scoop hurling out rocks and hoping at the same time their weight would not snap the line and throw rocks, catch and fishermen into the sea. "You never knew just how much was going to be 'the last straw'."

In twenty minutes of slow dredging a trawler could gather as much as one tonne of mussels.

As they began to make dredging pay the brothers were able to invest in a second, faster boat, the *"St. Vincent"*. Athol skippered this and his role was to go out and seek new mussel-fishing grounds. "He was always a better fisherman than I was," remembers Stuart, "more single-minded. I'd be sitting on the deck reading a book about engineering or teaching myself Japanese while he'd be studying charts working out new fishing areas."

Athol had indeed found a lucrative new crayfish ground about forty miles off the coast at North Cape; it covered an area fifteen miles long and two miles wide. It would need a new fishing method using 300 to 400 pots, and navigation by radar signals beamed off the land 30 miles away.

On his first trip out to see how efficiently the long line system worked, Athol chose a day with an adverse weather forecast. There was also a strong tide running. "North Cape is an eerie place," Stuart said. "The wind can howl for hours, then drop quite suddenly, leaving a flat calm. Daylight fogs drop down on you, severely limiting the visibility." Nevertheless Athol had radar on the *"St. Vincent"* and confidently made for the northern end of Ninety Mile Beach, an area exposed to buffeting winds that can come at one moment from the North-West, the next from the South-West. On this particular day the wind was North-East. "Athol anchored under a lee, preparing the long-line cray pot system to see if it was going to work. Then — without warning — the wind shifted around to the West.

"They went to start the *"St. Vincent's"* engines and the wiring suddenly shorted out. They tried to start them on the alternative battery, and — again — nothing. They were able to use the radio and they called us up on the mainland to tell us what had happened. The wind was swinging around," he continued, "and all the time the tide was getting lower. A line of surf could be seen coming out to the boat now, and it was at that point, I believe, that they should have cut her adrift and rode her through the surf then abandoned her."

When it was obvious to Athol and his two deck-hands that nothing could be done to save the *"St. Vincent"* they got into a rubber life raft and tried to keep clear of the surf and await a helicopter pick-up next morning. At the same time that Stuart McFarlane was frantically trying to get a rescue helicopter into the area, the life raft overturned and threw the three fishermen into the boiling sea. "One of the deck-hands got to shore, but was terribly knocked about by the surf. He died six months later. Athol and the other crewman's bodies were found some days later."

Stuart McFarlane and his father were shattered. The elder McFarlane had been saved a few years before from another trawler that had sunk beneath them and now the family had had enough. "I desperately wanted to get out of the fishing business," Stuart said.

He had a brief period away from the sea gathering fish pieces for a pet-food factory, but returned once more to trawl again on the *"Shenandoah"*. This time his luck had changed; he was able to perfect new methods of handling and processing fish, especially for the Japanese market.

* * *

In the back of his mind Stuart McFarlane had always believed there had to be an alternative to scratching at the ocean bed for the elusive mussel. The market was there; the mussel was diminishing. Why not *farm* it? Nobody had bred and collected mussels off the New Zealand coast, but there had been successful cultivation of other molluscs in other parts of the world. "I had always collected shells as a kid, and wondered about the fishes' breeding habits. Dad and I thought we should have a go.

"Shellfish do things for which we can offer no reason, but we accepted these things and worked around them. We built a small pontoon and hung Ti-tree branches underneath so they reached right down to the sea bed. It was now up to the spat — the tiny mussel embryos — to drift into the Ti-tree and fasten on to it. All we had to do was sit back and wait until they became big mussels."

To the McFarlanes' surprise, this was what happened. When they reckoned it was time to haul up the Ti-tree, the father and son were happily astonished to see it was heavy with fat, meaty mussels that filled nine sacks. "We considered that in two years we would be up and away as mussel farmers!" They were wrong. It took not two years, but eleven.

There were many unknowns, many pitfalls in the farming and harvesting of green-lipped mussels. What, for instance, would happen if you had large numbers of mussels — sixty tonnes for instance — hanging from one pontoon? Would they be too cramped and their growth inhibited? Would they run out of food? Would they be *happy*?

Allan McFarlane went off to Spain where they had been successfully farming the common blue mussel using the pontoon method, and when he returned the McFarlanes decided to build a large pontoon; it would be 140 feet long and 40 feet wide. And they believed they knew how to successfully 'spat' the ropes they would suspend beneath it. Explains Stuart: "An adult female mussel will exude 200 million to 300 million eggs when she is spawning. The eggs float about freely in the water in the chance they will meet sperm that comes from a male mussel in a white, seething mass that can turn an experimental tank of water so milky that it cuts down visibility to a few inches. The spawning is triggered by two factors: the water temperature and that state of fertility of the female. Fertilisation takes place in open water and for about 21 days the larvae are at the mercy of the currents. At this stage they undergo a metamorphosis for the last time, and become a mussel, having previously looked like 'half hinges' which could turn out to be scallops or barnacles. There is a vital period of 24 hours when they must find something to fix themselves onto, or fall to the bottom and die."

New Zealand's Fishing Industry Board, a quasi-government body, whose role it was to assist efficiency in fishing and the export of fish, were immediately encouraging to the McFarlanes. The Board helped with a grant of a couple of thousand pounds when the family decided to build the large pontoon, and the McFarlanes put in the rest. When it was completed and the Ti-tree brush in place, the cost had been £15,000. A storm hit the area six months later and the investment blew out into the wilds of the Tasman sea.

Stuart McFarlane now admits the pontoon was badly designed; wave action caused metal fatigue which they had not allowed for; secondly, they had mistakenly moored the pontoon in an area where the mussels sucked up a large amount of mud which inhibited their growth, putrifying them from the centre outwards.

The fishermen shrugged off their loss and 'walked away' from the pontoon. They would build another, smaller pontoon that could easily be moved around the coast, this time with mussels hanging from trailing ropes. The problem was how to actually fix the molluscs in place. After many hours at the drawing board at home, the inventive Stuart McFarlane found a way around the problem: inverted cones made of plastic. Their mesh would allow the sea — and spat — to flow through, but at the same time they would shelter the clinging mussels from strong buffeting from the current, and predators. Each cone would be suspended from ropes at short intervals.

* * *

A floating mussel fixes itself to an object in the sea by secreting a white liquid which becomes a hair-like thread the moment it makes contact with the water. The thread adheres to a rock — or in the case of farming — to a rope or cone. When it is only a quarter of an inch long, the mussel can use its tongue and thread to perambulate along the sea bed, moving at a rate of a gallop in 'snail terms'.

This time Stuart McFarlane made two pontoons, each 32 feet long. They were supported by tanks and each could keep afloat up to sixty tonnes of mussels. They were anchored in the path of strong tides and therefore escaped the clogging mud that had ruined the first harvest. Because of the turbulence of the sea in the area, each had to be moored by a pair of six-tonne blocks and three-tonne anchors; three tonnes of chain was needed to fix the blocks and anchor to a pontoon. Heavily spatted ropes were lowered from the pontoons and the McFarlanes went home to wait. At every anxious visit they were encouraged to see the mussels' growth-rate and the stability of the pontoons. But soon, yet another problem arose: *mussel rustling*. Because nobody can actually own a stretch of the sea, there are no proprietorial rights protecting a farmer's harvest. Consequently gangs who made raids on both pontoons were able to slash ropes and tow them away. "We anchored the *"Shenandoah"* near the pontoons a couple of times and fired shot-gun blasts over the heads of people hanging about the pontoons," says Stuart McFarlane. "But in the first year we lost about one hundred tonnes of mussels. All they had to do was open up about five big mussels and put them in a jar. They'd take them round the Auckland pubs and raffle them, getting up to $18 a jar. In one night an 18-foot boat could steal $2,500 worth of mussels without fear of being caught. It was as lucrative as robbing a bank, with much less chance of ever being grabbed."

Traditionally, the Maoris are the biggest consumers of mussels in New Zealand. The McFarlanes were supplying fat, meaty mussels to several Auckland fish-shops and restaurants and they were told the demand was insatiable. "We'd open at 6.30 a.m. when, later, we had our own shops," says Stuart, "and there'd be a queue of Auckland buses parked along the kerb. The Maori drivers were preparing to go on duty, but they had to have their daily 'fix' of mussels first. They all had their opening-knives in their belts and they'd swallow the fresh mussel raw before they got out of the shop."

The McFarlanes were not the only mussel-farmers in New Zealand; several other fishermen worried about the meagre catches from dredging were trying to perfect a farming technique in the Marlborough Sounds, a stretch of coastline similar to the Norwegian fiords. However without the plastic cone system — which Stuart McFarlane had cannily patented — their production was small.

* * *

Annoyed by the mussel poachers and worried that storms could wipe out their pontoons, the McFarlanes wanted to be more certain of fixing spat and systematically growing a harvest. Nature could be too unreliable. The Fishing Industry Board was unenthusiastic about breeding spat and being able to separate one tiny mollusc from another and fixing it to a growth medium. "In my usual rather stubborn way," recalls Stuart McFarlane, "I decided I could do it." He set up a small hatchery in his back yard and began experimenting.

"One morning in 1970, I had a phone call from the FIB. They said they would like to have some mussels to send to the United States and could I help them? They said there were medical experiments being undertaken on all kinds of shellfish. It was always Board policy to respond to requests because it could mean future exports. I gave them about 40 lbs. of mussels in a bag."

A month or two later, said McFarlane, Duncan Waugh, of

the Fisheries Research Division, was on the phone again. Could they have more mussels to send to the US? "The Company involved in the experiments was apparently excited about the results which indicated that an extract of the mussel gave relief to arthritis sufferers. Now they would like to have a couple of thousand juvenile mussels. Waugh promised to let me know what was happening."

Duncan Waugh did call again. This time, he said, he had two Americans with him and could he bring them out to see Stuart?

"They arrived with Duncan Waugh and he introduced me.

"Mr. Bob Gilmore, a short, stocky man, was introduced as President of the Aquaculture Corporation. His companion was an older man, a White Russian, marine biologist, a Dr. Loosanoff. He was a strongly-built fellow with a heavily-accented voice. He amused me by telling me that when he arrived in America he had been anxious to learn English, so he went off and worked in a lumber camp. When he emerged he discovered that what he had been learning for the past months was Norwegian; his fellow lumberjacks had all come from Norway. Dr. Loosanoff was now a scientist of some stature and had built a laboratory at Milford, Connecticut, for an offshoot of the National Aeronautics and Space Administration."

Stuart McFarlane remembers being astonished by one of Gilmore's first statements to him. "He said he might want to do business with me involving *millions of tonnes* of mussels.

"I got the feeling during the meeting that there was an atmosphere of condescension between us. After all, I was a fairly humble New Zealand fisherman." Nevertheless, enthused by the possibility of future orders for millions of mussels he still had to learn to breed, Stuart explained his problems so far. He still couldn't control spat, and until he could manage the juveniles it still wasn't a farming proposition, certainly not on a scale the Americans envisaged.

Loosanoff replied that he could breed oysters very easily in America and had been doing so for years to gauge the genetic effects of heavy metal pollution. Should McFarlane like to visit his laboratory he could arrange it.

In the meantime the FIB and the Ministry of Agriculture

were giving the visiting Americans VIP treatment. "A plane was laid on and they asked me to fly around with them looking for possible mussel-farming sites."

* * *

Stuart McFarlane recalls: "The Americans were talking about twenty square miles of farms! Computers would control the currents as they would be similar to the Mississippi; atomic power plants would provide the energy. And there was talk of purchasing obsolete aircraft carriers to be used as factories. The cost of it all would be in excess of $40 million. I felt that one of us must have been a little off-beam..."

Why would Gilmore and Loosanoff want to spend $40 million on mussel breeding? Surely Americans couldn't be persuaded to eat so many?

Then a vital word crept into the conversation: *cancer*. Medical tests had been taking place in the US to observe any possible use of extracts from molluscs that might have an effect on the world's most feared disease. "I was told that any American research agency only had to mention the word 'cancer' and they were hit with large amounts of money." During long discussions over dinner in Auckland restaurants (where Robert Gilmore showed bartenders how to produce an excellent martini) another medical word kept cropping up: *arthritis*. It was revealed that while the tests were going on in cancer wards, some patients who also suffered from arthritis reported that after consuming the New Zealand green-lipped mussel their aches and pains seemed to be relieved.

Robert Gilmore confirmed the advice given by Duncan Waugh and stated his interest in the mussel was as an arthritic treatment.

At this stage Stuart McFarlane was medically ignorant. He knew nothing of arthritis and its various forms, and would have been puzzled at the mention of the word 'placebo'.

The medical term 'placebo effect' was to haunt him, and to frustrate useful discussions between his own company and the medical profession about the mussel and its properties for years. Doctors had seen dozens of 'quack arthritis cures' come and go, with the patient the financial and sometimes physical loser. They understandably object to suffering people paying money they can often ill afford for a 'cure' that has no medical investigation or backing. *Any* tablet — made of sugar, flour, or even chocolate — can make some patients feel better immediately; basically because they want to feel better. It is the 'Placebo Effect'. The word 'placebo' comes from the Latin 'I shall please'. It can be a harmless capsule made from an inert substance; or it can be distilled water injected into the body with the promise that 'it will make you feel better'. Somewhere between 20 percent and 50 percent of patients in pain given a placebo will feel improvement — *for a time*. Their psyche has told their bodies to expect improvement and it comes. However it does not last.

Placebos are used in medical trials of drugs so patients and doctors can accurately gauge the effectiveness of a new treatment. The patient takes a placebo that exactly imitates the drug in taste and appearance, and then later he takes the drug, or the order is reversed. Only the chief tester in these trials knows which substance has been consumed first. Both patients and doctors are kept in ignorance of the identity of the substances until the trial has been completed.

* * *

By the time Robert Gilmore and Dr. Victor Loosanoff were ready to fly out of Auckland, a business accord had been reached. Stuart McFarlane believed he was on the brink of the most exciting period in his life.

(What happened to sour that relationship and lead to bitter written and verbal exchanges destroying any chance of the Americans and the McFarlanes working together, cannot at this stage be reported. Suffice to say a $5 million law-suit was launched by Aquaculture Corporation in 1982 against McFarlane and his company.)

CHAPTER THREE

THE VENTURE

The New Zealand magazine *"Commercial Fishing"* in October 1977, described how far Stuart McFarlane and his Technical Director John Croft had gone in his mussel-farming venture...

' Stuart McFarlane's mussel farming and processing operation in Auckland is the big success story of the New Zealand cultured shellfish industry,' it said.

'After 13 years of trial and error, Mr. McFarlane has perfected techniques for the controlled growth of *Perna canaliculus*, the New Zealand green-lipped mussel, and devised a process for extracting from the mussel meat a substance which has been hailed as a "wonder cure" by arthritis sufferers.

'Mr. McFarlane's industry is set to earn New Zealand millions of dollars in overseas exchange — probably the biggest single overseas export earner in the fishing industry. In April last year John Croft, McFarlane's technical director and a specialist in marine pharmacology, returned from the United States where he said he clinched a multi-million dollar export order for a million capsules a month for the first year, increasing 30 percent for the next five. That was the beginning.

'Today the North American market is just one of many overseas markets to which McFarlane exports in quantity. Trade with Australia grew at such a rate McFarlane Laboratories Pty. Ltd. was established in Melbourne, with branch offices in Sydney and Brisbane to handle sales and distribution. Offices have just been established in the United Kingdom and Hong Kong (John Croft flew in from there early last month to check on progress) and the company has its own distribution network in North America and Japan.

'But while it is all "go" on the McFarlane mussel farm and in the laboratory, and while all over the world the McFarlane product, marketed under (trade-name) is eagerly sought by those afflicted with painful rheumatics and arthritis, there is a certain irony to this success story: Mr. McFarlane told *Commercial Fishing* that he embarked upon the scheme of using the mussel meat as the basis of (trade-name) largely because his mussel farm would not show a profit if he marketed the shellfish for the table. And while (trade-name) is received with enthusiasm overseas, the extract is not viewed so by the New Zealand Health Department — which recently successfully prosecuted him for various alleged breaches of its regulations pertaining to marketing.

'In spite of the fact that in New Zealand Mr. McFarlane may make no claims as to the efficacy of his product in relieving the pain of rheumatic and arthritic sufferers (even though he has a file of literally hundreds of unsolicited letters from grateful users claiming various degrees of relief) (trade-name) has achieved a considerable standing by word of mouth and is sold in chemist shops throughout the country.

'Mr. McFarlane claims that the scepticism shown by the Health Department appears to have been extended to other Government agencies with regard to the provision of financial assistance for development. He recently made an approach to the Prime Minister, pointing out the overseas-earning potential of his product and seeking rationalisation.

'The Health Department did test (trade-name) on five people for a six-week period. The trial was made at Otago University by Professor T.C. Highton and Mr. A.W. McArthur. The results were published in March, 1975, in the *NZ Medical Journal*. The university team found the green-lipped mussel extract did not show any greater effect on the patients than placebos given in the same trial. Yet McFarlane showed an analysis of a trial in which definite improvements were shown by some patients.

'Meanwhile, (trade-name) samples have been sent to Germany, a secrecy agreement has been signed, and within a short time some of the expensive and time-consuming clinical tests necessary to validate the properties of natural extracts (Croft is adamant that (trade-name) is not a drug) will be completed and (trade-name) may be on the way to official recognition. If that happens, and the extract is accepted as a useful preparation for rheumatic and arthritic sufferers, it may be placed on the prescription list and made available to elderly sufferers at no cost. Meanwhile, (trade-name) costs $9.60 for 75 capsules.

'There is a certain sympathy in official circles for Mr. McFarlane's efforts to have the extract accepted by the Health Department. Health Minister, Mr. Gill, has said it is a pity (trade-name) is not under further investigation in New

Zealand. Claims by the United States company which first discovered that extracts from the green-lipped mussel had a remarkable effect in rheumatoid arthritis are supported by Duncan Waugh, director of the Ministry of Agriculture and Fisheries fisheries research division: "One member of my staff has tried a small amount and it does appear to have quite a remarkable effect," he said. "Her doctor was astounded at the sudden improvement in her condition."

'Mr. Waugh said the extract discovered by the American company was neither a miracle cure nor a drug.

'The McFarlane family was in the mussel business for many years before it ventured into farming the shellfish. With the steady depletion of the Coromandel and Thames mussel beds their operations were eventually confined to limited hauls by a solitary dredge. There were still odd pockets where private parties could get a feed — but they were inaccessible to commercial dredging.

'By then most of Auckland's mussels were coming from Nelson, where the beds were also being steadily depleted. The mussel population of the North Island west coast was then, as it is today, tremendous — but inaccessible to commercial dredging. And like the Nelson mussels, the west coast variety were smaller and darker than their east coast counterparts.

'Having conceived the idea of mussel farming the McFarlanes set about it, with the backing of the Fishing Industry Board. They set up a trial mussel farm in the Hauraki Gulf in the form of an enormous pontoon with the mussels growing on ropes trailing from it: "We worked on the assumption that we might be wiped out and have to start from scratch again," said Stuart McFarlane.

"'Indeed, we were wiped out, but the knowledge we gained from the experiment made it well worthwhile."

'The McFarlane's set up a new mussel farm between Waiheke and Pakatoa Islands, and eventually succeeded. Today they have six small pontoons measuring 22ft by 18ft, each supported by two cylindrical buoys (12ft long and 6ft in diameter, each with a 14-tonne lift) and one large pontoon, 70ft by 70ft. The smaller pontoons usually trail 80 22ft ropes, and the larger pontoon supports 400 26ft ropes. The tonnage of mussels growing on the ropes is far more than the pontoons would ever support on deck — because the green-lipped mussels weight only one sixth of their weight while in seawater.

'Spat is collected in the gulf by the company staff, taken to the laboratory and there fed on algae until it has grown to a length of about 3/4in., and grown to a length of about 6-8mm, in open seawater. That process takes about eight months. At that point the immature mussels are taken out to a farm and placed in PVC cones, inverted and strung on the ropes at 18in intervals.

'The cones, which were Stuart McFarlane's invention, contributed substantially to the success of his mussel culture programme. The immature mussels are placed in the bottom of the cone and as they grow they eventually fill the container, swelling and overflowing until they reach maturity and are harvested. The green-lipped mussels reach a length of about 15cm at maturity, and the meat weights between 38 per cent of their gross weight.

'Mr. McFarlane claims that he is achieving faster meat weight gains in the Hauraki Gulf than is being achieved in mussel farming operations in the Marlborough Sounds.

'Although he feared the depredations of snapper might reduce his harvest, in fact the mussels have been attacked only a few times by snapper, he said. Instead, the rafts have attracted a resident population — the patiki in particular — has a tendency to chase other fish species, including snapper, away from the mussels.

'Mussels are harvested twice weekly by the farm staff under foreman Chris Wedding, using the 55ft company launch *"Shenandoah"*. The ropes are hauled manually on to the decks of the pontoons and the cones emptied of mature mussels, which are placed in large plastic containers and taken back to the Fanshawe Street processing plant. For the most part, the mussels are grown on the ropes under the small pontoons, and then transferred to the large pontoon shortly before reaching maturity for a final fattening before harvesting.

CHAPTER FOUR

THE MEDICAL TRIALS

Medical trials of the mussel's efficacy had started. On 12 March 1975, the New Zealand Medical Journal carried a report of an experiment conducted by a team of Auckland researchers to gauge the effect of New Zealand green-lipped mussel extract on rats with induced polyarthritis (inflammation of several joints at the same time). The trial was conducted by Drs. J.C. Cullen, FRCS, FRACS; M.H. Flint, FRCS, FRACS and J. Leider, PhD, of the Department of Surgery, School of Medicine, University of Auckland.

The researchers explained as a preamble, that:

"During the last few months powdered encapsulated freeze-dried sections of New Zealand mussel (trade-name) has been introduced and sold in New Zealand as a health food. It has been suggested that this substance has a beneficial effect on different types of arthritis and patients taking the 25 day course have reported an improvement in their arthritic symptoms. However, objective assessment of improvement of patients with arthritis is difficult unless very large numbers of patients are involved. For this reason a study of the effect of (trade-name) on an induced experimental polyarthritis in rats has been carried out."

Twenty-eight albino rats — fourteen of each sex — had polyarthritis induced by the intradermal (within the skin) injection of freeze-dried, autoclaved microbacteria emulsified in paraffin. The single injection was given in the footpad. Swollen peripheral joints developed as a result.

The doctors described what happened next...

"Fourteen of the rats, seven of each sex, were fed on a normal laboratory pellet diet throughout the experimental period. The other fourteen rats were initially fed on a similar diet but immediately after the injection into the footpad they were placed on pellet diet to which freeze-dried mussel had been added. To obtain even mixing of mussel and pellet diet, 1g of the powdered mussel was added to 1000g of powdered pellet: the resultant mixture was moistened to form a thick dough and redried to strips to produce an equally acceptable pellet-type diet.

"The food consumption of each group was assessed daily to ensure that an adequate amount of the test material was being consumed. The rats were also weighed at the same time.

"The developing arthritis was assessed each day between the 14th and 28th days and thereafter three times a week until the end of the experiment at seven weeks. The arthritis score was assessed by the method of Zahiri, and others (1968), in which the severity was graded according to the number of joints affected in each paw. A maximum of five was given to those paws in which five or more joints were involved, excluding the injected paw a maximum arthritis score was therefore 15.

"The diet was taken equally well by both groups, there were no deaths in either group, nor was there any difference in body weights of the two groups during the experimental period.

"A florid polyarthritis with extensive joint involvement developed in all animals. Its severity was recorded in graph form, the total score for each group being divided by the number of rats to give an average figure."

And the final assessment?

"The induced arthritis used in this experiment (adjuvant arthritis) has been used as an experimental polyarthritis for many years. Its pathogenesis is uncertain but it is believed to be an immunologically induced disease either of a delayed hypersensitivity or of an autoimmune type (Jones, Ward, 1966). Although the disease is not rheumatoid arthritis it is similar in that the disease is predominantly of synovial tissue and affects many joints. This arthritis has been used for many years for drug trials when new drugs are introduced for the treatment of rheumatoid arthritis. In general, probably because of a similar pathogenesis in the two diseases, drugs which modify the inflammation in adjuvant arthritis also appear to have a beneficial effect on rheumatoid arthritis (Newbould, 1963).

"From the above experiment it is concluded that freeze-dried mussel does not have any beneficial effect on this induced polyarthritis in the rat and it is unlikely to have any effect on any other inflammatory arthritis of a delayed hypersensitivity or autoimmune type."

* * *

Does a rat with induced arthritis mirror the symptoms of a

human being with the real disease?

John Croft in his book 'Relief from Arthritis', discusses the difference between the effect of the mussel extract on human beings with real arthritis and the *inflammation deliberately induced* in animal subjects.

He says:

'During experimental work with the mussel extract preparation on animal subjects it became evident that this substance worked in a manner which was different from that of the usual anti-arthritic drugs. In very generalized terms, the mussel extract gave different results in trials with animal subjects to those produced by synthetic drug preparations.

'The results were such that it might just be that the extract is attacking the cause rather than the effect of the arthritis! The expression "just might be" has to be emphasised because as yet no definite proof exists to clarify the possibility. What could stimulate such a dramatic thought?

'It is based on the speculation that, as the standard anti-inflammatory treatments are known only to attack the effect of the disorder, *i.e.* the inflammation, and as the extract does not appear to attack the inflammation directly, then it may be that the mussel is penetrating below mere symptoms to the cause itself... in trials using rats in which inflammatory conditions 'similar' to those found in arthritic conditions are created in the animals, these are inflammatory conditions, and they respond to treatment by anti-inflammatory drugs, but they are not of arthritic origin. They do not respond to treatment with the mussel extract, which suggests that the extract does not possess direct anti-inflammatory properties. However, inflammatory conditions which *are* of arthritic origin *do* respond to treatment with the mussel extract...'

In the same 1975 issue of the New Zealand Medical Journal there appeared a report of a 1974 'pilot study' on the mussel's effect on *humans* with arthritis. It was sponsored by the Medical Research Council of New Zealand and was undertaken by Dr. T.C. Highton, FRCP, FRACP, Associate Professor the Department of Medicine at the University of Otago, Dunedin, New Zealand, and Dr. A.W. McArthur, MB, Dip. Clin. Pharmacol., a medical research officer at the same unit.

It was a finding which was to bitterly anger the producers of the mussel extract for the brevity of the experimental period and the number of arthritics taking part.

The doctors said in their introduction:

"Following an initial approach in the standing committee of therapeutic trials of the Medical Research Council and subsequent accounts in the lay press to the effect that the New Zealand green mussel might be of value for its remedial properties in rheumatoid arthritis, the rheumatic diseases unit of the department of medicine agreed to undertake a preliminary trial to enable a decision to be made was to whether a major multi-centre trial on this product was warranted.

"This product is marketed by McFarlane Laboratories Auckland under the name (trade-name). Sufficient material in capsule form for oral administration was supplied for the treatment of six patients together with a similar quantity of placebo which was virtually indistinguishable in physical appearance and smell.

"The form of the trial was a typical double blind cross over trial with randomised allocation of order to either 'active' or placebo capsules for six weeks treatment on each. The trial period of six weeks was chosen because it had previously been stated that there was often a three week delay in the appearance of beneficial effects.

"Entry was by informed consent from a group of patients who had rheumatoid arthritis for periods varying from one year to 20 years while one patient had suffered for two months only. All patients were enthusiastic to participate in the trial. Severity of the disease ranged from multiple joint involvement with all the criteria of active disease to one patient who had relative restriction of movement and pain in two joints only. All patients had symptoms and signs which were potentially reversible by therapy. Thus it was considered that this fairly wide range of disease activity would permit easier detection of any beneficial therapeutic effect of the test compound. Five of the six patients were female.

"Those patients on maintenance gold or low dose steroids continued with this regime but anti-flammatory drugs were withdrawn 14 days before the commencement of the trial to allow for a 'washing out' period. Patients were permitted paracetamol tablets for analgesia, the number of tablets ingested serving as one of the indices of the pain experienced.

"Standard assessments of the subjective and objective

patient responses were made after the wash out period at the beginning of the trial and fortnightly thereafter.

"A Ritchie articular index of joint tenderness was drawn up on a 0-3 scale assessing each joint for tenderness while the number of swollen joints was also recorded. Accurate measurements of joint range of movement and joint circumferences were recorded. Joint swelling was estimated and recorded on a 0-3 scale.

"Estimation of strength of grip, recorded after the average of three attempts was derived using a standard modification of a sphymomanometer cuff. The time to walk 10 metres was measured by stop watch in the usual standard manner.

"At each clinic attendance, consultation times being at the same time of the day throughout the trial, laboratory checks on haematology, note book records of patient assessment of morning stiffness duration, pain experienced each day on a 0-4 scale, and the number of paracetamol tablets needed daily were noted and recorded.

"Clinical assessment of response, patient well-being and patient preference for each type of drug at crossover and at the end of the formal trial were recorded.

"Five patients completed the trial. Assessment on the basis of the Ritchie Index indicated that joint tenderness was greater in four patients when on (trade-name) and greater in one when on placebo. Four patients experienced improvement in the joint swelling scores on (trade-name) while in one the scores were worse. Grip strength was greater in one on (trade-name) and less in four while morning stiffness was less in three and greater in two. Patient discomfort was less in one, greater in three and unchanged in one on (trade-name). There were fewer tender and swollen joints in three on (trade-name) and more in two. Sedimentation rate was higher and more paracetamol was taken by all five patients completing the trial while the time to walk 10 metres was greater on (trade-name) in two patients and less in two.

"This pilot trial involved a small number of patients only. The subjection of patients suffering from a serious disease such as rheumatoid arthritis to trial with a new therapeutic substance can only be conscientiously undertaken when there is a reasonable expectation of success. However, the patients that were involved in this study underwent a most detailed evaluation of their articular state during the trial according to the most rigorous criteria for rheumatological assessment and it is considered that the results give a reasonable indication of the expectation or otherwise of success with a larger trial. The results of the pilot study have not been such as to warrant extension to a larger group or to substantiate claims made for the material in the lay press. In the event some of the patients did deteriorate during the course of the pilot trial: one refused to continue soon after crossover (from the placebo) because of the deterioration in her condition and was subsequently admitted for intensive therapy."

If McFarlane Laboratories had believed that research was going to bestow to the mussel the blessing of the medical world, they now realised that would be a long way off.

Then came a light at the end of the tunnel — shining 13,000 miles away...

CHAPTER FIVE

THE GIBSONS

In the early 1960's, at Belvedere Hospital, Glasgow, Scotland, Dr. Robin Gibson was helping to deal with an outbreak of croup among young children. It worried him and the other medical staff involved, that few were responding.

For some time, Gibson, a dedicated man in his 30s, had been reading about homoeopathic remedies and the claims made of cures in cases where conventional medicine had failed. (Homoeopathy is a method of treating disease by prescribing minute doses of drugs, which in maximum dose, would produce symptoms of the disease.)

Dr. Gibson decided to treat one of his croup patients with a homoeopathic remedy he had been reading about. Within hours the child had recovered, the only one to make such rapid progress. It was the final evidence Gibson needed to make his mind up to specialise in homoeopathy. It was at a time when fewer 'orthodox' medical men were practising the science, even though there were, and still are, excellent hospitals in the United Kingdom devoted to its use. "It wasn't easy," recalls Robin Gibson. "My colleagues and friends thought I'd gone a bit cranky. But I was becoming increasingly frustrated by conventional medicine administered for some diseases and the more I studied, the more I realised that homoeopathy had just as much to offer as orthodox medicine."

By 1965 Gibson was treating patients on a part-time basis at the Belvedere Hospital while he studied immunology — the workings of the body's immune system — and allergies at the Western Infirmary in Glasgow.

Seven years later an event occurred that was to change his life: a Trident aircraft crashed on take-off at London Airport and among those killed was the consultant physician at the Glasgow Homoeopathic Hospital. Gibson's interest in the science and his immunological background was known among his colleagues and he was offered the position, which he quickly made up his mind to accept.

In the meantime, his wife, Sheila, had graduated not only as an M.D., but as a B.Sc. in biochemistry. She was working as a resident consultant at the Western Infirmary and at the Stobhill Hospital, specialising in gynaecology and researching genetic diseases. She had decided it was time to leave the posts to have their children, Sandy and Catriona. When they became of school age, Sheila Gibson joined her husband in his homoeopathic work at the Glasgow Homoeopathic Hospital.

* * *

The Glasgow Homoeopathic Hospital, founded in 1880, is a cheerful, bustling treatment centre housed in a solid Victorian mansion at 1000 Great Western Road, which adjoins the main road from Glasgow to the airport, about three miles from the city. In the last century, the building had been the residence of a prosperous Glasgow merchant. Today the hospital is administered by the Glasgow Health Board and is part of Britain's National Health Service. Its staff of five doctors — the Gibsons and three others practising conventional medicine — work on two floors on which there are 30 beds. Each year they see about 30,000 outpatients and treat them at the Homoeopathic, or at two other associated clinics in another part of Glasgow. Arthritic diseases of all kinds account for about third of all cases, the rest being made up of heart conditions, asthma, multiple sclerosis, ear, throat and nose complaints, and a wide spectrum of allergies.

When we were there a few days before Christmas, lights from a giant Christmas tree were reflected in the highly-polished entrance-hall floor. Patients were sitting on beds playing cards, reading, watching television, hobbling painfully about on crutches, or manoeuvering wheelchairs.

Dr. Robin Gibson, 50, a stocky, taciturn man with dark hair flopping across his forehead, explained his hospital's activities. Reserved, with a dry sense of humour after his initial reticence has been put aside, Gibson makes it clear from the outset that he had been wounded by the attitude of his medical lords — the powerful Medical General Council — and is wary of drawing their ire a second time.

His wife, Sheila, neat and shapely even in her white medical coat, has blue eyes that sparkle with vivacity and is less constrained. They met in 1959 at Glasgow University and today live a few miles from the hospital growing and eating pesticide-free fruit and vegetables, each a healthy example of the diet-consciousness they are always preaching.

It had been in 1971 that the couple had on their appointment list one morning a Miss Christina Gardiner, aged 83, whom they had been treating for osteoarthritis. Unfortunately after many months, she had gained no relief from her disease despite all the homoeopathic and conventional treatments she had been given.

This morning, however, the courageous Miss Gardiner had something to tell the doctors...

* * *

A friend of Miss Gardiner's, living in Auckland, had been reading in the newspapers of the consumption of capsules of freeze-dried New Zealand green-lipped mussel by arthritics. They claimed they were eating them and getting relief from their pain. She had bought a bottle and airmailed it to Miss Gardiner in Glasgow.

Arriving at the clinic, the elderly spinster asked the Gibsons whether she should try out the 'cure'.

Robin Gibson read the label on the bottle, took out the capsules and noticed a fishy smell; then he asked Miss Gardiner if he might break a couple open to analyse them. She agreed.

Dr. Gibson said: "They were simply a whole food and could not possibly do any damage, so I told her to go ahead. I did not put any great store by the (trade-name) pills at this stage. My view was that they could not do any harm and might give a psychological boost to Miss Gardiner if nothing else."

Miss Gardiner went home and took her capsules as directed — three a day. When she returned for her regular check-up the Gibsons found a surprising improvement in her condition, remarkable enough in their eyes to cause Dr. Robin Gibson to write off to McFarlanes in Auckland asking if he might have further samples to test. He received them almost by return airmail.

At best Dr. Gibson had expected a psychological improvement in his patient — the Placebo Effect. But her gain was now outlasting the usual remission brought about by hope, and her condition was creating such interest among the medical staff and her friends that she became — in the Gibsons' words — 'a bit of a celebrity'. She joined a local arthritics' association and talked about the capsules, and soon she became the association's chairman. (It was on her way to one of the meetings in 1980 that she was struck by a car and killed.)

* * *

The Gibsons were now giving the New Zealand green-lipped mussel extract to other arthritics and they were so sure they were getting results that they decided on a properly conducted trial, using patients with well-documented case histories as guinea pigs.

Robin Gibson warned McFarlane laboratories that this would be no quick look at the mussel — it could take *several years*.

McFarlanes air-freighted packages of the encapsuled mussel powder to Glasgow and the Gibsons put themselves on a course of it for six months, to be certain there were no harmful side-effects.

Forty-six out-patients attending the Glasgow Homoeopathic Hospital were chosen as test subjects. Their condition satisfied the American Rheumatism Association diagnostic criteria for 'classical' rheumatoid arthritis: all had been given conventional 'front-line' anti-inflammatory drugs and when they had not responded, had been given homoeopathic treatments. They had either failed to improve on either treatment and their condition was static, or they were getting worse.

The arthritic guinea-pigs were asked: "Would you like to try a recently discovered treatment?" An arthritic will grasp at most straws offering hope and they said they would. However the doctor assured them that none of their drugs would be discontinued, they would keep on with their therapy, whether orthodox or homoeopathic.

Assessment of the severity of arthritis depends to a great extent on how much pain and discomfort the patient says he or she is feeling. But the physician can use several methods of gauging how crippling the disease is without relying too much on the sufferer's self-diagnosis of pain intensity. A patient can be timed walking a certain distance, grip-strength can be accurately measured, limbering-up time recorded. The Gibsons would parallel their own observations and tests with the patients' assessments, and improvement would only be considered to have occurred if both patient and physician agreed and if there was objective evidence (like walking against the stop-watch) to suggest it.

The doctors were aware that on average, at least one third of people who visit surgeries are 'placebo reactors' — given any tablet, they will feel better for a short while at least.

While the trials were proceeding there would be laboratory tests on blood-counts, serum biochemistry and serology when the trial began, then fortnightly for six weeks and monthly thereafter.

Ten osteoarthritis patients, all showing x-ray evidence of bone wear and tear were chosen for the tests.

The Gibsons drew up a list of questions for each patient to answer which would give the researchers an accurate idea of their functional ability before and after taking the mussel extract.

After each question they asked about the degree of ability.

"Can you turn your head from side to side?"

(Answer: yes, with no difficulty/yes, but with difficulty like pain, stiffness or weakness/No.)

"Can you comb your hair at the back of your head?"
"Can you close drawers (with arms only)?"
"Can you open doors?"
"Can you lift a full teapot?"
"Can you lift a cup with one hand to drink from it?"
"Can you turn a key in a lock?"
"Can you cut meat with a knife?"
"Can you butter bread?"
"Can you wind a watch?"
"Can you walk?"

"Can you walk without
  (a) Someone's help?
  (b) Crutches?
  (c) A walking stick?

"Can you walk up a flight of stairs?"

"Can you stand up with your knees straight?"

"Can you stand on your toes?"

"Can you bend down to pick something up off the floor?"

"Do you have energy?"

The 46 rheumatoid arthritis patients were aged between 23 and 71 years. They had each had arthritis with symptoms severe enough to ask for medical help. Their disease span ranged from one year to 24 years with a mean of 7.6 years.

At the end of the long trial the Gibsons passed their verdict on the New Zealand green-lipped mussel...

- 34.8% of the patients who had taken it had improved 'considerably'.
- 32.6% were helped, but to a lesser extent.
- 32.6% were not helped at all.

Of the 10 patients with osteoarthritis who had been taking the mussel extract, three were suffering from general osteoarthritis, *i.e.* in many parts of the body, one had two joints affected (both hips), and six had only one joint affected — either a hip or a knee.

The three patients with general osteoarthritis improved; no significant improvement was observed in the six patients with single-joint osteoarthritis, or the patient who had two joints affected.

The Gibsons observed that no patient in either the rheumatoid arthritis group or the osteoarthritis group had been able to discontinue the mussel therapy completely without experiencing some set-back, but it was possible that some of the patients might be able to discontinue taking it in the future.

One important finding was that nine patients — eight with rheumatoid arthritis and one with osteoarthritis had been able to discontinue all other therapy and were taking the mussel extract alone.

The doctors had closely watched for toxic side-effects from the mussel and observed that five of the test subjects had initially felt slight nausea when they had started taking the mussel extract, but in most cases this had appeared to settle down within two or three weeks. Nine patients reported flatulence and some loosening of the bowel, but that had also settled down when the dosage was reduced. Three patients told the Gibsons that their stiffness had got *worse* for the first ten days and one patient had experienced prolonged stiffness which only disappeared when the dose was reduced to a single capsule a week. No other side-effects were reported.

* * *

Having recorded the facts, the doctors now interpreted them so that doctors reading their papers in medical journals would have their considered opinion of the therapeutic work of the sea creature.

"The results of this preliminary study," wrote the Gibsons, "indicate that the extract of the green-lipped mussel was beneficial to two-thirds of the patients with rheumatoid arthritis... the improvement was independent of the age of the patient and the duration and severity of the disease.

"This was encouraging, as all these patients were failing to maintain improvement on both conventional first-line anti-inflammatory agents and homoeopathy. Some were deteriorating. The next stage in management of these latter patients might have involved consideration of one of the second-line drugs... (like) levamisole or corticosteroids... which are associated with a high incidence of toxic effects.

"The extract of this shell-fish would therefore seem to be both reasonably effective and safe. In a condition such as rheumatoid arthritis in which the patient is often taking drugs constantly over a long period of time, this is not without its advantages."

They went on:

"The results of this present trial are in sharp contrast with the results obtained by Highton and McArthur[*] who reported no improvement in 6 patients in a double-blind cross-over trial conducted over a period of only 1 month. Their trial, however, can be criticised on several counts. Firstly all previous anti-inflammatory therapy was stopped for a period of 2 weeks prior to the trial, and over the period of the trial,

---

[*] The Otago trial.

Paracetamol being substituted. This would inevitably produce a worsening of the disease. Secondly, the patients were on green-lipped mussel for 2 weeks only, which in our experience is insufficient time for any significant therapeutic effect to be observed. The patients in the present trial began to show improvement only after 3-4 weeks in most cases. Only a few showed improvement earlier than this. Experience in Glasgow has shown that at least 6 weeks is required to assess Placebo Effect. In this connection it is interesting that of the 15 patients in Group III, 8 showed an initial improvement which lasted 4-5 weeks only, and was considered to be merely placebo effect. Thirdly, the number of patients in Highton and McArthur's trial was far too small to make any proper assessment.

"In a trial which commenced a few months prior to the green lipped mussel trial, in which 95 patients with rheumatoid arthritis satisfying the same criteria were followed up for a year, 41 on salicylate therapy, and 54 on homoeopathy, only 6 of the patients on salicylate were satisfactorily controlled. The other 35 had dropped out of the trial either because they failed to be adequately maintained or because of unacceptable side effects. Although the 6 patients who remained on salicylate felt that they had not deteriorated, their mean values for articular index, limbering up time and grip strength were in fact worse than they had been at the beginning of the trial. The patients in the salicylate group who remained in the trial were those who were least affected by their disease. The patients on the green lipped mussel on the other hand, were more severely affected, having failed to respond to all previous orthodox anti-inflammatory treatment. It can be seen... that green lipped mussel, either alone or in combination with other first-line anti-inflammatory treatments, was much more effective in the control of rheumatoid arthritis than was salicylate alone.

"This initial study was not double-blind and both the patients and the physicians knew what was being given. A rigorously controlled double-blind study is now under way and the results will be reported later.

"In contrast with the results obtained in the patients with rheumatoid arthritis, the results in the patients with osteoarthritis were poor. Only 30% were helped. The numbers, however, were small. It is interesting that the patients with generalised osteoarthritis tended to benefit whereas those with single joint osteoarthritis did not. This perhaps highlights a basic difference between generalised osteoarthritis and single joint asteoarthritis. 'Perna canaliculus' is believed to have an anti-inflammatory effect. It may well be that the generalised form of osteoarthritis in common with rheumatoid arthritis is primarily an inflammatory disease while single joint osteoarthritis may have a different aetiology as far as the pain is concerned.

'In conclusion, it would seem that this extract from the New Zealand mussel 'Perna canaliculus' is a safe and effective alternative therapy in rheumatoid arthritis and in some forms of osteoarthritis. The safety and efficacy will be further evaluated by means of a double-blind trial."

* * *

In addition to their trial findings, the Drs. Gibson had x-ray photographs showing a phenomenon thought to be unique in the annals of medicine: *reconstitution of a diseased arthritic hip.*

The x-rays were taken of Mrs. Jean Wesley. Dr. Robin Gibson sent them to *The Lancet* and other medical journals with this accompanying letter on 30 January 1980:

'The Editor,
The Lancet,
7 Adam Street,
LONDON WC2N 6AD
Sir,
JOINT REGENERATION IN RHEUMATOID ARTHRITIS

Rheumatoid arthritis contines to be a major cause of morbidity and loss of working days in this country. Despite many recent additions to both first and second line treatments, approximately two thirds of rheumatoid patients experience a progressive deterioration in health which seems not to be reversible by standard pharmaceuticals.

Six years ago we began trials with a freeze-dried extract of Perna canaliculus, the New Zealand green lipped mussel. In a double-blind trial, this material produced clinical improvement in 70% of patients with rheumatoid arthritis, and 40% of those with osteoarthritis. We now have data on over 400 patients. A number of these have experienced an almost complete reversal of their clinical symptoms. The following case history is only one of a number of such cases but is worth reporting because of the striking x-ray changes which have occurred.

CASE REPORT

Mrs. J.W., aged 59, first presented with rheumatoid arthritis 16 years ago at the age of 43. She was seen at the Centre for Rheumatic Diseases in Glasgow, and despite treatment with many anti-inflammatory drugs, experienced a progressive downhill course. Five years ago she was seen at the Orthopaedic Department of the Victoria Infirmary for assessment for surgery to a completely ankylosed left hip. Surgery, however, was postponed and in June 1979 she presented at the Rheumatology clinic of the Glasgow Homoeopathic Hospital, seeking further non-surgical help.

By that time she had been unable to walk without two elbow crutches for the preceding 8 years, and had been confined to a wheel-chair on several occasions. She was completely unable to perform any housework, and had been granted a mobility allowance and a permanent home help. She had been on corticosteroids for 7-8 years but these had been terminated a year prior to being seen at the Homoeopathic Hospital. Her articular index (AI) was 38, limbering up time (LUT), 60 minutes, grip strength in each hand 50mm. of mercury, functional index (FI) 26 and pain on the visual analogue scale 90%. Her Hb was 11.6 G% and R_3 was positive, 1/16.

She was put on to Perna canaliculus extract, 1050 mg/day, and when seen two weeks later was already feeling less stiff and sore. Over the next 7 months she experienced a steady improvement and full movement gradually returned to the left hip which she had not been able to move for at least 5 years.

When seen for assessment on 10 January 1980, she was feeling very fit. AI was 4, LUT 5 minutes, grip strength in each hand 200 mm. of mercury, FI 3 and pain on the visual analogue scale 10%. Haemoglobin was 13.6 G% and R_3 was negative.

She has been walking without the elbow crutches for the past 3 months and only takes one in case of need when walking long distances, because of residual pain in the left knee and right ankle. X-ray performed on 10 January 1980 showed complete regeneration of the left hip joint with reconstitution of the articular surfaces and joint space. X-rays of both hands and wrists are also showing some improvement. We will continue to monitor this and will report the results in future studies.

As far as we can discover, x-ray evidence of reversal of pathological changes of this order in rheumatoid arthritis has not previously been reported. After 6 years' study we are of the opinion that the use of this extract of the New Zealand green lipped mussel is a major advance in the treatment of rheumatoid arthritis. The case reported here shows that the body's capacity for renewal and regeneration is much greater than is currently accepted by most medical practitioners, and that the outlook in this crippling disease need not be as pessimistic as many of us are led to believe.

Robin G. Gibson, M.R.C.P., D.C.H.
Sheila L.M. Gibson, M.D., B.Sc.
T.N. Cowle, M.D., B.Sc., F.R.C.R.

Department of Clinical Pharmacognosy,
Glasgow Homoeopathic Hospital,
Glasgow G12.

The x-ray photographs and letter were returned to the Gibsons. The Editor of *The Lancet* declined to publish them.

* * *

Two years after the x-rays had been taken of her hip, we spoke to Mrs. Jean Wesley, now 62, asking if it was possible that her x-rays had been mixed up with another patient's?

"There is no way," she said. "The x-rays were taken *twice*, just to make sure. And I was shown them at every stage. I have a copy of them in my house and I impress all my friends with them. A doctor in Canada, like many people, did not believe that my hip had been miraculously cured and I have sent him copies of my x-rays to prove it."

Mrs. Wesley said she had suffered from crippling rheumatoid arthritis for 16 years and for eight years she had only been able to walk with the aid of elbow crutches. She had to spend long spells in a wheelchair and was unable to use her hands properly. Her husband, a textile company representative, would take her around in his car with him every day because he was afraid to leave her alone in case she fell or spilled hot liquids on herself.

In 1975 she went to Glasgow Infirmary where he left hip was x-rayed. *It showed complete fusion of the joint.*

"They wanted to give me a replacement joint," said Mrs. Wesley, "but as this had not worked with my mother I refused to have it done. But I was suffering.

"I had heard about Dr. Gibson purely by chance. My own doctor was ill and someone suggested I should try the Homoeopathic Hospital. I didn't have much hope because I had suffered so long and I wasn't getting any younger. Dr. Gibson treated me with (trade-name) as an outpatient and after about five months I gradually began to be able to do things I hadn't been above to do for years.

"The first thing I noticed, was that one morning, without thinking, I lifted up the teapot. I hadn't lifted a tea *cup* for over twenty years! My hip gradually became easier and I was able to swing it freely and walk properly. I could hardly believe it! It seemed like some sort of miracle. Dr. Gibson took x-rays in 1980 and I don't think he could quite believe it either when the x-rays showed that the hip had healed. But the x-rays — and the way I feel now — prove it. I don't need crutches any more and I can walk normally at home without my husband worrying. The only time he takes me with him now is when I want a ride in his car. I still take three mussel tablets a day. I wouldn't dare do without them. The only snag is the increasing cost. I feel strongly that (trade-name) should be available of the National Health. So many old-age pensioners suffer the way I used to do, and they can't afford to buy (trade-name)"

CHAPTER SIX

A MEDICAL BONUS

As if it were not enough for arthritics to have pain, the large amounts of anti-inflammatory drugs they need to take to quell it often results in severe irritation of their stomachs, even ulceration.

Dr. K.D. Rainsford, of the Biochemistry Department, at the Medical School of the University of Tasmania, Hobart, Tasmania, and Dr. M.W. Whitehouse of the Department of Experimental Pathology, John Curtin School of Medical Research, Australian National University, Canberra, resolved to study the mussel extract and any *gastro-protective* qualities it might have in addition to its anti-inflammatory potential.

The doctors starved male and female rats for 24 hours and then allowed them water before the experiments. The animals were dosed orally with mixtures of acetylsalicylic acid (aspirin) and mussel preparation and it was discovered that they developed 'much less gastric mucosal damage than animals given ASA (aspirin) alone.'

They pointed out: "Since gastric ulceration and haemmorrhage frequently occur with ingestion of ASA (aspirin) and related non-steroid anti-inflammatory drugs, it seemed that there may be real therapeutic benefits (with respect to the gastric mucosa) by adding the mussel preparation to (aspirin) using it as a pharmaceutical adjunct."

The scientists also experimented on pigs by giving them drugs alone and drugs with mussel extract.

Their findings: "These data indicate that unlike many potential gastroprotectants this mussel preparation does not impair, but rather reinforced the therapeutic activity of low doses of either ASA (aspirin) or indomethacin (a common analgesic used for arthritic pain). These observations were confirmed by data from using several different batches of the mussel preparation harvested at different times. The relative specificity of this mussel preparation was indicated by parallel experiments with equivalent quantities of similar freeze-dried preparations from other New Zealand shellfish, namely oysters, scallops and paua, which all failed to afford gastroprotection when co-administered with ASA (aspirin)".

The doctors then sounded a final note of caution... "that the results of these studies of protection by lipid fractions against NSAI drug-induced ulceration may be unique to the rat."

In other words, the results could only be regarded as providing *suggestive* evidence as a basis for possible investigation in man.

* * *

In September 1980, Drs. Robin and Sheila Gibson, along with Drs. Valerie Conway M.B., Ch.B. and David Chappell F.R.C.S., from the Victorian Infirmary, Glasgow and the Department of Clinical Pharmacognosy, Glasgow Homoeopathic Hospital, published in *The Practitioner* the result of further comprehensive trials of the mussel extract on human beings.

During the largest trial yet conducted they had set out to evaluate the efficacy of the preparation more fully. It would be a double-blind trial and was designed this time to include a greater number of patients suffering from osteoarthritis so they might obtain a more accurate assessment of the effects of the agent on the symptoms of that disease.

Sixty-six patients were chosen for the trial. 28 of them suffered from classical rheumatoid arthritis and 38 had clinical and radiological evidence of osteoarthritis.

All patients were on the waiting list of the orthopaedic unit of the Victoria Infirmary, Glasgow, for joint surgery.

All patients were taking some form of non-steroidal anti-inflammatory therapy for their disease. They were told they would be taking part in a double-blind trial to 'assess the value of a new anti-inflammatory preparation'. All agreed to co-operate. The doctors asked them to keep taking the drugs which had been prescribed for them without alteration. They would consume the trial material as an additional treatment.

In Auckland, McFarlane Laboratories had prepared 350 mg. mussel extract capsules for the test, and at the same time, capsules of powdered fish that were identical in appearance, taste and smell to the mussel preparation, which would be given to the patients as a *placebo i.e.* they were pharmacologically inactive.

When they arrived in Glasgow both lots of capsules were handed to the hospital pharmacy department where they were coded so that the identity of the 'active' and 'inactive' preparations would be unknown to both doctors and patients. Previous tests on patients by the Gibsons had shown that the effects of the mussel extract could remain in-evidence for two to three weeks after the cessation of therapy and this ruled out the possibility of a full double-blind crossover trial.

For three months the arthritic patients took their randomly allocated double-blind therapy, after which their condition was assessed. Then they were given what was known to be actual mussel extract for a further three months, thus making sure all the patients had consumed the test material.

The codes were not broken until the patients had been in the trial for six months and neither the patients nor the physicians conducting the trial knew whether there had been any actual change in therapy in the second three-month period.

The patients went before the team of doctors at monthly intervals at the orthopaedic outpatient department. With the exception of joint movements which were measured at the initial visit, then at three months and six months, full clinical assessments were made at each visit. Any previously unnoticed side-effects were also recorded.

For *rheumatoid arthritis* patients checks were made on:
- articular index of joint tenderness
- morning stiffness (limbering up time)
- grip strength in each hand
- pain
- functional efficiency
- the time taken to walk a measured distance of 50 feet.

The patient and the physician made their own assessments of whether or not there had been any improvement, and the patient was only considered to have improved if both the patient's and the physician's opinion agreed. Additionally, there had to be objective supporting evidence of improvement.

For *osteoarthritis* patients, progress was assessed on:
- degree of morning stiffness (limbering up time)
- pain
- functional efficiency
- the time taken to walk 50 feet
- the range of movement in hip and knee joints.

Again, only if there was agreement between patient and doctor on improvement was improvement registered.

The doctors' final verdict after breaking the codes:

"Of the 66 patients in the trial, eight dropped out before the end of the first three months — three had rheumatoid arthritis and five had osteoarthritis. Three of these patients were admitted to hospital for reasons unrelated to their arthritis, two had difficulties with transport, one had previous dyspepsia and felt the capsules disagreed with her, and two gave no reason.

"Ten of the 17 rheumatoid patients on the active preparation improved during the first three months compared with three of the 11 patients on the inert preparation. In the osteoarthritis group six of the 16 patients on the active and three of the 22 patients on the inert preparation, improved. During the second three months of the trial, a further six rheumatoid and six osteoarthritic patients improved. At the end of six months, therefore, 19 of the 28 rheumatoid patients (67.9%) and 15 of the 38 osteoarthritic patients (39.5%) felt that they had benefited from being included in the trial. If the patients who dropped out are disregarded, as in most instances the reason for drop-out was unrelated to the arthritis, then 76% of the rheumatoid and 45% of the osteoarthritic patients improved.

"Of the 66 patients in the trial, 46 suffered from night pain. This was relieved in 17 patients on active treatment and in two on placebo — a 37% response to the active preparation.

"Apart from the patients who improved when assessed objectively, seven patients, four on placebo and three on the active material, showed a temporary response lasting less than two months. Since previous experience with rheumatoid patients in Glasgow has suggested that a placebo effect is not maintained for longer than six weeks these patients were classed as placebo responders.

"Six patients experienced an increase in the severity of their symptoms two to four weeks after starting active treatment. This exacerbation lasted for one to two weeks, after which they made good progress. It is interesting that a similar flare-up has been observed in other patients one to five weeks after beginning treatment with this extract (Croft, 1979).

"SIDE EFFECTS: Apart from the exacerbation of symptoms nine of the 66 patients in the trial experienced side effects, eight on the active preparation and one on the inert material. Two patients experienced increased stiffness which disappeared within two to three weeks. One patient had epigastric discomfort, one suffered from increased flatulence and four, of whom one was on placebo, had nausea. One patient retained fluid which was reversed by stopping the treatment for a week and recommencing at a lower dose level.

"DOSE ADJUSTMENT: When patients were seen to be well-maintained on the active preparation for two months or more, an attempt was made to reduce the dose. It was found that several patients could be satisfactorily maintained on two capsules (700 mg.) per day."

The doctors went on:

"It was encouraging that the proportion of patients who responded to treatment with the mussel extract in the double-blind trial was similar to that obtained in the preliminary study, 67.9% of rheumatoid patients and 39.5% of osteoarthritic patients benefiting from this form of therapy. The measures of pain, stiffness and the ability to cope with the environment improved significantly in those patients who responded to the therapy. Grip strength did not improve significantly in the short-term double-blind trial although in the pilot study, which included a number of patients with less severe destruction of the joints of the hands, there was significant improvement in strength. Many of the rheumatoid patients in the double-blind trial had marked deformities of the hands and had difficulty in grasping the cuff of the grip-strength apparatus. It was therefore not surprising that no marked change was seen in this measure. There were no significant changes in joint function as assessed by measurement of the range of movement in the osteoarthritic group as a whole although individual patients did improve. This again was not surprising since gross destructive changes requiring joint surgery are unlikely to be reversible by drug therapy.

"Most of the patients in the study were old and had suffered from their disease for many years. The mean ages were 68.8 and 57.0 years, respectively, for osteoarthritic and rheumatoid patients and from their disease for many years. The mean ages were 68.8 and 57.0 years, respectively, for osteoarthritic and rheumatoid patients and the mean duration of disease 12.9 and 17.8 years, respectively. All patients were severely affected and all had deteriorated to the stage where they were on the waiting list for joint surgery for the relief of pain and disability. They were therefore patients who were nearing the end of the road as far as orthodox therapy was concerned. While it is unlikely that many will have been improved to the extent that joint surgery becomes unnecessary, nevertheless the quality of life for about half of them had been improved considerably. The encouraging fact that improvement could be obtained in such old and long-standing cases confirmed the impression gained from the preliminary four-year study that the benefit was related neither to age of the patient nor to the extent or severity of the disease.

"Toxic effects were uncommon and, with the exception of the one patient who retained fluid, were mild. The mussel extract used in the present trial was as effective as gold, though not as effective as levamisole in improving pain, stiffness and grip strength. The drop-out and side-effect rates moreover were much lower with *Perna canaliculus* than with either gold or levamisole. These latter are both second-line drugs with a high incidence of toxic reactions. It is therefore suggested that *Perna canaliculus* may prove to be a safe alternative to second-line drugs when first-line treatment is failing to maintain the patient in a reasonably comfortable and functional state.

"The dose of mussel extract required to maintain improvement varies from patient to patient. In the four-year pilot study it was possible to reduce the dose in a considerable number of patients to one capsule per day or less after they had been on the therapy for a period of several months. In the double-blind trial some patients managed to reduce their dosage from three capsules (1050mg) per day to two capsules (700mg) per day without experiencing any set-back. None has so far been able to reduce the dose further, but none has yet been on the therapy for longer than six months.

"In conclusion," said the doctors, "the trial suggests that the extract of the green lipped mussel, *Perna canaliculus* is an effective supplement or possible alternative to orthodox therapy in the treatment of both rheumatoid arthritis and osteoarthritis. It reduces the amount of pain and stiffness, improves the patient's ability to cope with life, and apparently enhances general health. Added to these benefits is the low incidence of side effects. It would therefore seem that this substance could be of considerable value to patients suffering from these two chronic and disabling conditions."

* * *

Exhilerated by the success of their trials the Gibsons flew out to New Zealand to see for themselves the farming and harvesting of the New Zealand green-lipped mussel. They expressed enthusiasm to Stuart McFarlane, and when an Auckland newspaper heard of their visit, agreed to an interview. They recounted the results of their trials and repeated the story of the x-ray evidence, without revealing the name of their patient.

When they got back to Glasgow they opened their mail. There was a scolding communication from the General Medical Council, the highest medical disciplinary body in Britain: their newspaper interview 13,000 miles away was considered to be 'advertising for business'. They were ordered to write an apology.

* * *

Understandably, both doctors are today unwilling to again risk provoking the General Medical Council. However Robin Gibson feels he must defend allegations — from even his fellows at the Homoeopathic Hospital — that his evidence of the efficacy of the mussel is inconclusive. "We were amazed at what the x-rays showed. We could hardly believe it ourselves. It just shows we (doctors) don't know everything. It *did* happen. And we still have the x-rays to prove it."

In early 1983 Sheila Gibson was planning a follow-up investigation of forty patients who have been treated at Roundelwood Centre, at Crieff, Scotland, by she and her husband for the past five years. Some of these have been using the mussel extract alone for their arthritis, but the majority have been given a three-pronged treatment of the mussel, physiotherapy and a wheat-free diet. Her results will be presented to 'The Practitioner', 'The Lancet' and other medical journals.

Since their trial evidence was published in 'The Practi-

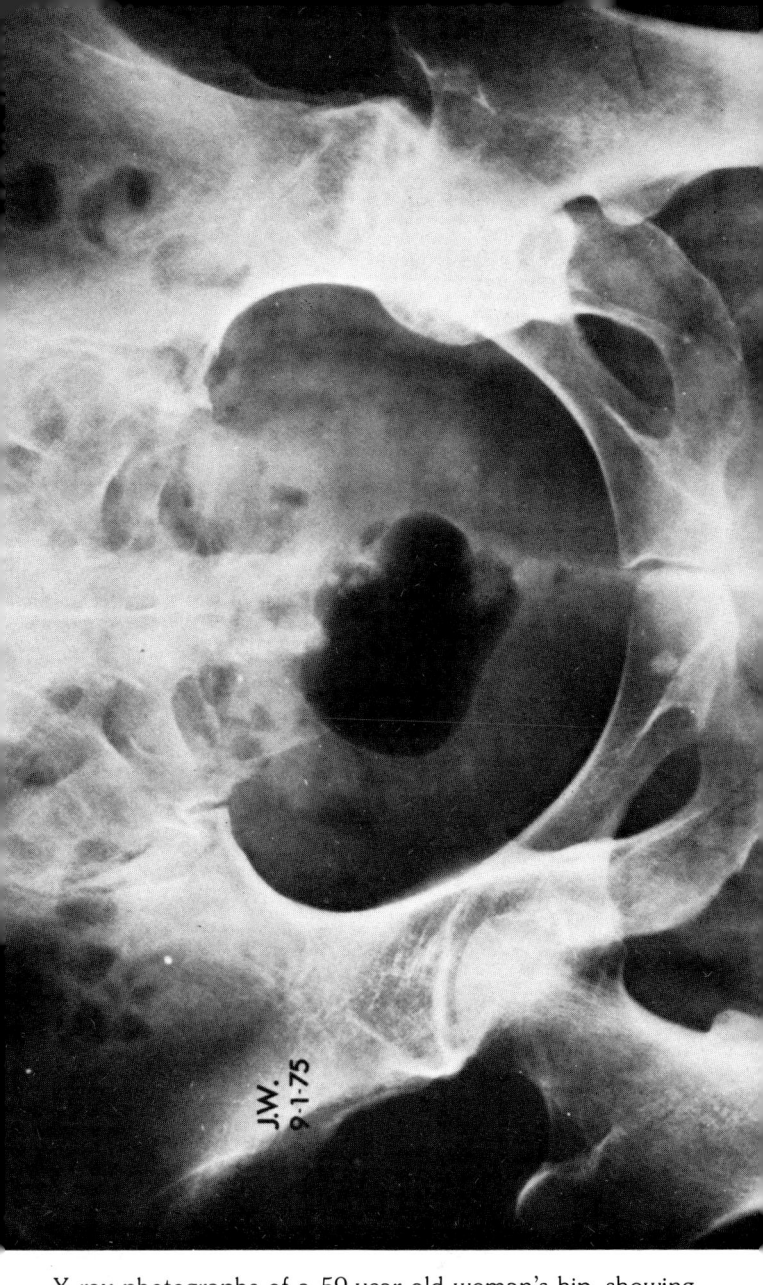

X-ray photographs of a 59-year-old woman's hip, showing its condition before taking the green-lipped mussel extract.

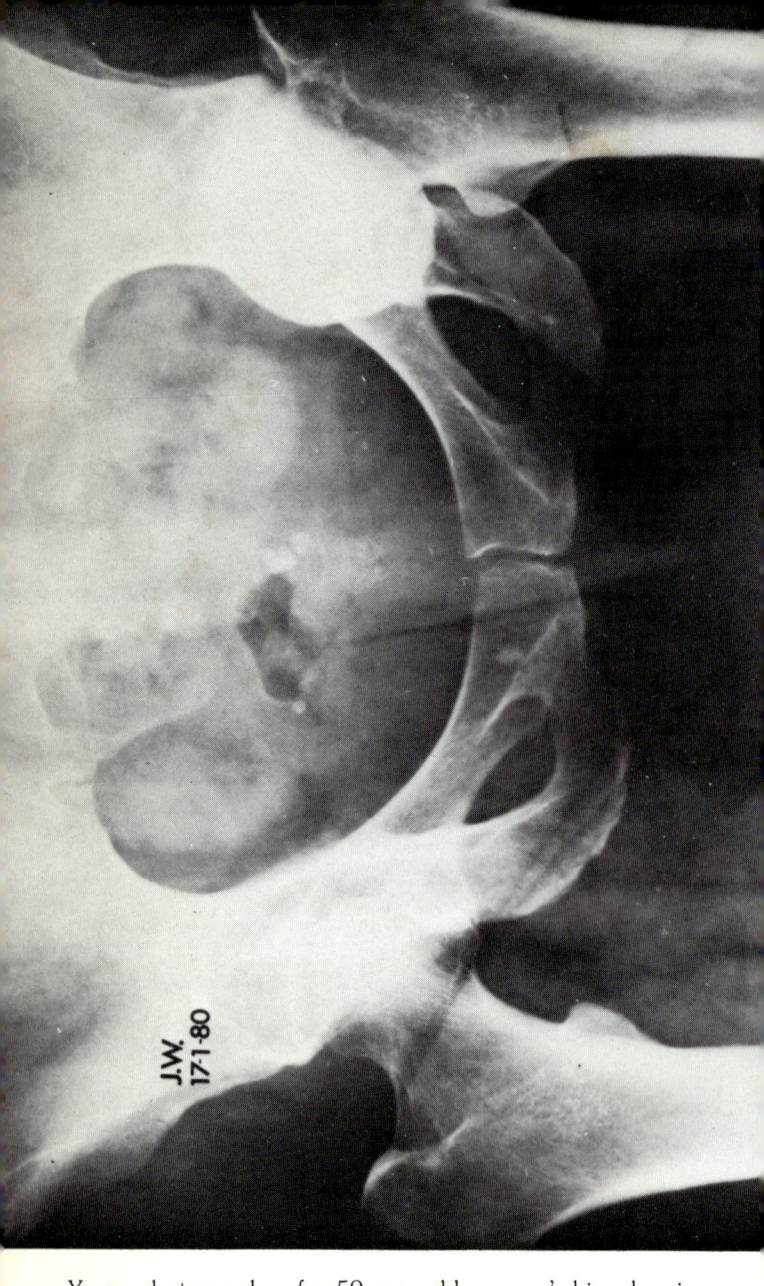

X-ray photographs of a 59-year-old woman's hip, showing its condition after taking the green-lipped mussel extract.

tioner'[*] twenty doctors from around Britain have written enquiring about the New Zealand mussel.

* * *

In May 1982, Mrs. Dorothy McGregor, aged 67, was carried into the treatment rooms at the Homoeopathic Hospital. For three years she had been bedridden and her hands were so swollen and distorted her husband, Thomas, had to feed her. She was admitted for five days for tests and told to take the mussel capsules and go on a strict diet that was wheat-free and banned barley and pork. Four weeks later she walked up the hospital steps with the aid of two sticks.

* * *

When the Gibsons prescribed the mussel extract for 32-year-old farmer James Mitchell, of Blairlinnen, near Glasgow, he initially regretted having gone to see them. He took the capsules and felt *worse*. "I'd developed rheumatoid arthritis in the joints of my hands in 1979 and they became so painful I could not work on the farm and was unable to drive a tractor. I was considering giving up farming altogether.

"I was willing to try anything and was put on (trade-name) by Dr. Gibson. But instead of getting better it became much more painful. Dr. Gibson told me it was normal, and doubled the dose. Then, about six months after starting the treatment, I suddenly began to get better. Within weeks I was able to do everything on the farm again — including driving the tractor. Now I'm just a normal farmer. I have the odd twinges in my wrists and knee joints but after what I experienced it's nothing — probably just old age setting in!

"I don't take any treatment at all now, but I have plenty of (trade-name) handy, just in case."

* * *

In 1981 two doctors at the Department of Medicine at the Auckland Hospital, Auckland, New Zealand, Dr. Thomas E. Miller, M.Sc., Ph.D., Research Fellow, and Dr. Douglas Ormrod, A.I.S.T., Research Assistant, reported that they had tested the New Zealand green-lipped mussel on rats deliberately given arthritic symptoms.

[*] In 1981

A carrageenan (a seaweed extract used for testing anti-inflammatory agents)-induced inflammatory swelling of the rat hind footpad had been used as the experimental model. Non-steroid anti-inflammatory agents were introduced and were shown to have the power of reducing the oedema (swelling).

The doctors explained the experiment...

Animals were anaesthetised with ether and laid on their stomachs in front of the operator but facing away. The feet were held by the toes and 0.1 ml of carrageenan solution, held in a warmed syringe was injected subcutaneously into the footpad. Footpad thickness was measured using an engineer's pocket thickness gauge (No. 7308, Mitutoyo Mtg. Co., Japan). The gauge was modified by reduction of the spring tension and surface area of the striker. Detectable swelling was demonstrable two hours after challenge and reached a peak four hours after challenge. Most of the swelling had subsided by 24 hours. In these experiments, measurements of footpad thickness were made before the injection of carrageenan at two, four and sometimes six hours later.

The preparation of *Perna canaliculus* was supplied as freeze-dried powder available commercially. For injection the powder was ground further in a Krupps domestic coffee grinder. This was suspended in saline at a concentration of 100 mg/ml and administered either into the peritoneal cavity using an 18G needle or by gastric gavage (tube feeding).

Aspirin, phenylbutazone and indomethacin were used as "control" agents with recognised anti-inflammatory activity and were prepared as follows — *Aspirin:* Soluble aspirin was dissolved in distilled water so that a dose corresponding to 200 mg/kg was administered in a volume of 1 ml. *Phenylbutazone:* A suspension of phenylbutazone in 1% carboxy methyl cellulose (CMC) was prepared. The concentration was such that 1 ml. administered to a rat corresponded to a dose of 200 mg/kg. *Indomethacin:* A dose of 5 mg/kg was given in 1 ml of 1% CMC.

Because, explained the doctors, the mussel extract was a crude preparation, some delay in absorption could be expected. A highly significant reduction in the footpad swelling was seen two hours after administration in a group of animals given the mussel or aspirin. Four hours later the anti-inflammatory effect of the mussel extract was more effective than aspirin, although aspirin itself still markedly reduced the inflammatory response.

One concern the doctors had was that the observed results with mussel extract might be a non-specific response. So two related materials — one the residue from a chloroform extract of a preparation of *Perna canaliculus*, and the other a sample of fish processed in the same way, were tested under strictly monitored conditions. No anti-inflammatory acitivity was demonstrated.

Later the doctors performed a large experiment using 104 animals. They found that the active material in the extract had a cumulative effect. They then assessed the power of the extract given to the rats by force-feeding them through tubes. They discovered that the administration of the extract by the gastric route for a period of 14 days did not produce any reduction in the footpad swellings.

The doctors concluded: the mussel extract was shown to have a 'marked' anti-inflammatory effect on the swellings. "The experiments have shown that the active agent was rapidly absorbed after intro-peritoneal administration and there was evidence of a cumulative effect. No anti-inflammatory activity could be demonstrated however when (the extract) was given orally, even after repeated administration.

"Although," they went on, "(trade-name) is marketed widely and subjective reports of individuals who have benefited from the material have been published, few experimental investigations have been carried out. In one study, adjuvant-induced (a substance used to aid other drugs) arthritis in the rat failed to respond to prolonged oral administration of (the extract), but as no known anti-arthritic agents were included for comparison the significance of the observation is difficult to assess. We too, using a different model, have been unable to demonstrate an anti-inflammatory effect after oral administration of (the extract) and it may be that the oral route in the rat is inappropriate. The results of a recent double-blind clinical trial have shown that (trade-name) taken orally, can be of benefit in rheumatoid and, to a lesser extent, osteoarthritis in man.

"At this stage it is not possible to equate the anti-inflammatory activity demonstrated in the present experiments with the putative (reputed) therapeutic effects of (the extract) and more appropriate models will need to be developed. The results, however, provide and encouraging start by characterizing some of the pharmacognistic properties of the material and detailed studies are currently being carried out to identify the active agent."

* * *

Later in 1981, four researchers, from the Department of Medicine, and Postgraduate School of Obstetrics and Gynaecology, at the University of Auckland, decided to set up a trial which would aim to clear up disputed aspects of previous findings on the efficacy of the mussel extract.

Backed by the New Zealand Medical Research Council two Research Officers, R.A.F. Couch, Ph.D., and D.J. Ormrod, B.Sc., and two Research Fellows, T.E. Miller, Ph.D., and W.B. Watkins, Ph.D., drew up the parameters of the trial. They would concern themselves with claims that had been made that it may be helpful in the management of inflammatory joint diseases — claims that had been supported by one clinical trial and rejected by another.

Animal studies, they pointed out, using the rat footpad oedema model had shown that the preparation possessed moderate anti-inflammatory activity when taken orally. Activity had also been demonstrated when the preparation was injected intraperitoneally, but this report had been challenged on the basis that the anti-inflammatory activity could have resulted from counter irritation. The possibility would be examined.

* * *

Female rats from an inbred Dark Agouti strain were selected for the trials. An inflammatory oedema (swelling) was produced by the subcutaneous injection of carrageenan (the derivative from seaweed traditionally used to test anti-inflammatory drugs), into the plantar region of each hind footpad. Freeze-dried New Zealand green-lipped mussel, scallop and oyster, all collected from the same area of the Hauraki Gulf near Auckland were made into solutions, so one substance's action on the swellings could be compared with the others.

The scientists found: "Oral administration of the (mussel) material... did not affect carrageenan-induced oedema." The intraperitoneal route (injecting into the peritoneal cavity) was used initially. "This raised the possibility of counter-irritant effects complicating the interpretation of the results.

"The problem was addressed directly and it was found that while unfractionated and partially fractionated material did induce some counter-irritancy, most of the oedema reducing effect was due to a genuine anti-inflammatory acitivity... furthermore the anti-inflammatory property was confined to extracts of the green-lipped mussel and could not be demonstrated in similar preparations from other molluscan bivalves.

"The experiments have shown that *Perna canaliculus* does contain an anti-inflammatory macromolecular moeity which acts through mechanisms other than counter-irritancy. The activity has been concentrated in a two-step fractionation procedure and there is evidence that the active material is either a protein or is protein associated. Finally, the anti-inflammatory property is species associated. The results are encouraging and form the basis for further research into the chemical nature of the material and its therapeutic prospects."

* * *

It was early in 1981 that three researchers at St. Bartholomew's Hospital in London decided on a four-week trial on fifty arthritic outpatients to test the anti-flammatory power of the New Zealand green-lipped mussel.

They put up a notice in the Department of Rheumatism clinic waiting-room inviting patients to take part in the trial, naming the product which had by now received wide media publicity.

The team was Dr. E.C. Huskisson, consultant physicain, and two clinical metrologists, Ms. Jane Scott and Ms. Rachel Bryans. Their trial was supported by a grant from the Arthritis and Rheumatism Council.

Dr. Huskisson reported several months later in the *British Medical Journal* that his team had used a placebo capsule consisting of dried fish which 'had an offensive smell indistinguishable from that of (trade-name).' During the crossover trial, each treatment was added to the patients' existing drug regimen. All patients had arthritis that was adequately controlled by existing treatment, and all had requested a trial course of the new mussel product. During the trial the staff noted the pain intensity, duration of morning stiffness, articular index etc., and the patients' preference for one or other treatment.

Twenty-six patients completed the study. It was found that 10 patients had preferred the mussel extract, nine preferred the inert fish in the imitative capsule and seven had no preference. 13 out of 22 patients (59%) with morning stiffness at the start of study noted a substantial reduction in its duration, and in two cases it disappeared completely. *Figures for the placebo group were identical.* "One patient was so enthusiastic," reported Dr. Huskisson, "about the first period of treatment, that she returned her stick to the physiotherapy department; she was receiving a placebo."

Three patients stopped the treatment because of side-effects while taking the mussel product. One had headaches; one abdominal pain, diarrhoea and headaches; and one constipation. Additional minor side effects were reported by patients receiving the placebo.

The researchers summed up:

'These results show clearly that a single couse of (trade-name) was not superior to a fish extract in rheumatoid arthritis. Previous evidence for the effectiveness of (trade-name) is slender. The anti-inflammatory activity shown by Miller and Ormrod was obtained by intra-peritoneal and not oral administration. Intraperitoneal administration of chemicals may have a spurious anti-inflammatory effect and is therefore unreliable. The effects in patients shown by Gibson *et al* were slight. Their study remained double-blind for only three months, during which time 10 out of 17 patients with rheumatoid arthritis receiving (trade-name) improved compared with three out of 11 receiving placebo. The difference is not statistically significant. The results of measurements of pain, stiffness, and articular index were not given for patients receiving placebo, and no other evidence was put forward to show that (trade-name) was superior to placebo.

'A four-week course of (trade-name) does not appear to be worth while except for the very considerable placebo effect that any new treatment has in rheumatoid arthritis.'

* * *

When they read their copy of the *British Medical Journal* Drs. Robin and Sheila Gibson were stung by what they felt was its unfairness to them and to the product. They wrote to the journal and their letter was published in May 1981:

'Sir,

In reply to the article by Dr. E.C. Huskisson and others about (trade-name), an extract of the green-lipped mussel *Perna canaliculus* in rheumatoid arthritis (25 April, p 1358), we would like to make the following comments.

1) To our knowledge, no physician has claimed that one month on (trade-name) has any obvious effect on the majority of arthritic sufferers, and the term "course" on the bottle is, in our opinion, misleading. Like Dr. Huskisson, we did not find a noticeable difference between the active preparation and the placebo at the end of one month. The numbers of patients improving on the active treatment, however, increased with time and, although not reaching significant values by three months, were significantly different by six months. If Dr. Huskisson had wished to reproduce our trial conditions, it is difficult to understand why he carried out his double-blind study for only one month instead of three.

2) We agree that the placebo figures are not tabulated for the three-month period in the trial report. This occurred because the tables were shortened and simplified for publication. These data are now presented for the active and placebo groups of rheumatoid and osteoarthritic patients in the table. These show that articular index, limbering-up time, and functional index all improved significantly in the rheumatoid group on active treatment and that pain as assessed by the visual analogue scale, functional index, and the time taken to walk 50 ft (15 m) improved significantly in the osteoarthritic group on active treatment. No significant improvements were obtained in any parameter in either placebo group.

3) Prior to carrying out the double-blind trial, we had had

over five years' experience with (trade-name) and had noted that on discontinuing this substance patients could maintain improvement for periods ranging from several days to several months. For this reason, a complete double-blind cross-over trial over a short period is unlikely to provide useful information as patients receiving placebo in the cross-over period may still be benefiting from the active substance given in the first period of the trial.

4) It is pertinent to re-emphasise that the group studied in our trial was somewhat atypical in that all the patients were on a surgical waiting list, having deteriorated to the stage where joint surgery was considered necessary. The average age was high, 56·7 years for the rheumatoid patients and 69·0 years for the osteoarthritic patients. Many of them were over 70 years of age. None had heard of (trade-name) and all believed that only surgery could help them. This contrasts with Dr. Huskisson's group, all of whom had heard of (trade-name) and had actually asked for this treatment. They thus entered the trial with high expectations of success. This in itself could account for the high proportion of placebo responders and it decreases the objectivity. Experience in Glasgow has shown that in rheumatoid arthritis the placebo effect is unlikely to last for longer than six weeks. This, coupled with the fact that (trade-name) can take from one to three months to have an effect means that, in our opinion, a double-blind trial should last for at least three months. Moreover, the dose used in this trial was 900 mg/day compared with 1050 mg/day in our study. Some patients require even higher doses and may need to alter their dietary habits (unpublished data).

We have been using (trade-name) for over seven years and have found it *to be the safest and most effective preparation for both rheumatoid arthritis and osteoarthritis* that we have yet come across. The title of Dr. Huskisson's study "(Trade-name) is ineffective in rheumatoid arthritis", is misleading in that it differs from his concluding remarks that (trade-name) is ineffective when given for only one month. It is unfortunate that such a valuable addition to materia medica could be misjudged by this title.

Robin G. Gibson
Sheila L.M. Gibson

Glasgow Homoeopathic Hospital
Glasgow G12 ONR

If Robin and Sheila Gibson believed at the outset their trials with the mussel capsules would interest their medical colleagues, they were to be disappointed. Sheila Gibson says: "The trouble is that there is a lot of bitchiness at the top of our profession. Although it is now generally recognised that many homoeopathic remedies *do* work, any trials, or discussions referring to them are still looked upon with great suspicion. Their attitude is if *they* don't know about these advances they can't be happening...

"The (trade-name) trials were, in their minds, associated with yet another 'quack' homoeopathic remedy, particularly as at the time of our trials it wasn't possible to explain exactly what it was in the mussel that was leading to the dramatic results thrown up in our trial. Now that Paul Gregory" (a scientist at the Royal Melbourne Institute of Technology) "has been able to isolate the precise acids and chemicals in the mussel that are proving so beneficial, further trials are likely to get more recognition.

"There is no doubt in our minds that if our research had been done by conventional physicians in a conventional hospital, rather than by homoeopathic doctors in a homoeopathic hospital, it would have been given far wider recognition. But even if they didn't quite believe us, surely there was enough evidence provided by us to at least initiate a full-scale investigation and double-blind trials over six months or a year instead of the trivial and inconclusive trial carried out at St. Bartholemew's Hospital by Huskisson.

"We are bitter about the reception of our trial because we are convinced that (trade-name) can be greatly beneficial to large numbers of arthritic sufferers, particularly if it is taken with physiotherapy and a wheat-free diet. We, of course, are continuing to give our patients (trade-name), but we worry about the millions of other arthritic sufferers around the world who are being denied the benefits of (trade-name) because of the short-sightedness of the medical Establishment. (Trade-name) will eventually be recognised as an important aid to treating arthritis. But meantime, patients have to suffer."

* * *

As the McFarlanes' executives scanned the medical journals of half a dozen countries for reports of trials on their mussel extract, they were stopped in their tracks by a report in *The Medical Journal of Australia*, of 9 August 1980.

Under the heading 'Reports of Cases', three Adelaide doctors reported that the mussel extract (they published its trade-name) had caused hepatitis in a woman aged 64. They wrote:

"GRANULOMATOUS HEPATITIS
AND (MUSSEL EXTRACT)
M.J. Ahern, M.B., B.S., F.R.A.C.P., M.R.C.P.
S.C. Milazzo, M.B., B.S., F.R.A.C.P.
R. Dymock, M.B., B.S., F.R.C.P.A.
The Queen Elizabeth Hospital, Adelaide.

"Granulomatous hepatitis developed shortly after a patient with mild chronic polyarthritis started taking (mussel extract), a proprietary product. No other likely cause for her liver disease could be determined.

"(Mussel extract) is a proprietary product said to be derived from the New Zealand green-lipped mussel. It has been extensively promoted in Australia and elsewhere in magazines, radio and television, and in a paperback publication, as being beneficial to people with arthritis. We report the occurence of granulomatous hepatitis in a woman who was taking this substance.

"CLINICAL RECORD

A 64 year old woman presented in July 1979, with a three week history of colicky pain in the epigastrium and right hypochondrial region, which was associated with anorexia and malaise. One week before presentation she had noticed jaundice. For five years the patient had suffered from a non erosive seronegative symmetrical polyarthritis affecting wrists and metacarpophalangeal joints, and had taken indomethacin (75 mg day) regularly during this period. In May 1979, she started taking (mussel extract) (two tablets a day). She took no other medication and did not abuse alcohol. The pain in her joints had diminished with the onset of jaundice. There was no pruritus.

"On admission to hospital the patient was jaundiced but no signs of chronic liver disease were evident. The liver had a normal span, was palpable 2cm below the right costal margin, and was tender. Examination of the cardiovascular, respiratory and central nervous systems showed no abnormalities. The joints appeared normal, apart from some soft tissue thickening of the metacarpophalangeal and proximal interphalangeal joints. The serum bilirubin level was elevated to 112 pmol/L (conjugated bilirubin, 89 pmol/L), alkaline phosphatase level to 381 u/L, aspartate aminotransferase to 69 u/L and gamma glutamyl transferase to 553 u/L. The erythrocyte sedimentation rate (Westergren) was 99 mm in one hour. An abdominal sonogram demonstrated a well visualized gallbladder with no calculi. There was no evidence of dilated intrahepatic ducts, and the pancreas was not enlarged. A percutaneous 'thin needle' cholangrogram failed to show opacification of the biliary ducts. Hepatitis B surface antigen was not detected, and the liver spleen nuclide scan was normal.

"A liver biopsy was performed, and this revealed moderate distortion of the hepatic lobules exhibited numerous epithelioid granulomata with giant cells and focal necroses. The changes of granulomatous hepatitis were also apparent within the portal tracts. The presence of eosinophils associated with the granulomata was in keeping with a drug reaction. No microorganisms were either seen on microscopy or were cultured.

"All medications were stopped on admission to hospital. The patient was discharged two weeks later, feeling well and with improving liver function as indicated by the following serum levels: total bilirubin, 52 pmol/L, alkaline phosphatase, 272 u/L, aspartate aminotransferase, 46 u/L, and gamma glutamyl transferase, 310 u/L. One month after discharge from hospital her bilirubin level was normal, alkaline phosphatase level was 136 u/L and gamma glutamyl transferase level was 67 u/L. After three months all tests of liver function gave normal results, and the erythrocyte sedimentation rate had fallen to 18 mm in one hour.

"DISCUSSION

There was neither clinical nor radiological evidence to support a diagnosis of sarcoidosis. In addition, it is unusual for uncomplicated sarcoidosis to be associated with elevated alkaline phosphatase and aspartate aminotransferase levels, also jaundice is rare, and most of the cases of jaundice due to hepatic sarcoidosis which have been reported have been in North American Black patients.

"Granulomas in the liver have also been recognized in

association with a variety of infectious diseases ranging from viral to rickettsial and spirochaetal infections, and as reactions to a number of drugs, including phenylbutazone, allopurinol, sulphonamides, methyldopa and hydrallazine. The spontaneous resolution of this patient's illness, and the results of investigations, substantially excluded the presence of tuberculosis, brucellosis, lymphoma, primary biliary cirrhosis, infectious mononucleosis, gytomegalovirus and Q fever.

"The patient was taking only two medications before her illness, indomethacin and (mussel extract). Indomethacin has been implicated as a cause of centrilobular necrosis, and of cholestatic hepatitis but to our knowledge, not of granulomatous hepatitis. Furthermore, there had been no indication in this patient of any adverse reaction to indomethacin during the preceding five years. She had started taking (mussel extract) three weeks before the onset of jaundice, and continued to take it until her admission to hospital. The temporal relationship of the onset and resolution of the disorder with the ingestion of (mussel extract) suggests that this substance was the cause of the granulomatous hepatitis. Rechallenge with (mussel extract) was considered, but was rejected on ethical grounds."

In the same journal, two months later, John Croft wrote from Auckland:

GRANULOMATOUS HEPATITIS AND (MUSSEL EXTRACT)

Madam: I read with interest the recent case report regarding the suggested involvement of (mussel extract) in the development of granulomatous hepatitis.

"While accepting the facts as reported, several aspects of the interpretation of the case history are arguable and several alternative conclusions could be drawn from the information reported.

"Two products were in fact taken concomitantly by this patient and one of these (indomethacin) has been proved to hepatotoxic. (Mussel extract), on the other hand, has been widely used since 1974 by an extimated 750,000 people. So far, there have been no reported incidences of liver dysfunction associated with the use of the substance. Why, then, was (mussel extract) selected as the causative agent?

"It could certainly be argued that only a small proportion of the group members were also taking indomethacin in conjunction with (mussel extract) selected as the causative agent?

"It could certainly be argued that only a small proportion of the group members were also taking indomethacin in conjunction with (mussel extract). However, even if one proposes a figure of 5%, it indicates 37,500 people in this category making the apparent adverse combination of extremely low incidence.

"On the basis of the information available the involvement of (mussel extract) in so far as the least favourable conclusions in relation to this product have been made, leaving other equally valid conclusions apparently unconsidered.

"In this regard a more objective and appropriate heading to this case report would have been 'Indomethacin, (Mussel Extract) and granulomatous hepatitis'.

"From the point of view of logic one wonders how it is that a single unfavourable effect of an agent becomes publishable material whereas any attempt to publish a favourable report, supported by an equivalent amount of data with the inherent uncertainties, would surely have been rejected (quite rightly so) as lacking scientific proof.

J.E. Croft

23 Heather Street
Auckland, New Zealand.

Dr. Milazzo replied:

"Madam: I comment on points raised in the letter from J.E. Croft.

"The paucity to date of reports of adverse effects associated with the use of (mussel extract) may reflect a lack of adequate machinery for surveillance and reporting of such associations when they concern a preparation that is freely available without prescription, and often consumed without the knowledge of the attending doctor. In our case, it was only after searching inquiry into possible provocative agents had been pursued, and after the nature of her illness had been revealed by biopsy, that the patient disclosed that she had taken (mussel extract) for three weeks before the development of granulomatous hepatitis.

"It is a widespread misconception among lay people that substances derived from 'natural' souces are likely to be innocuous. Claims by the promoters of such products that they possess particular (and invariably beneficial) biological activities fail to alert most people to the likelihood that, at least in some individuals, and in certain doses, adverse effects may well occur.

"In contrast to the now sophisticated systems administered by health authorities for multistage precautionary assessment and monitoring of newly introduced pharmaceuticals, proprietary biological products, even in a concentrated form, can be marketed without undergoing exhausive safety testing and without an early warning system being available for detecting idiosyncratic adverse reactions.

"As our report stated, it seemed likely that (mussel extract) was responsible for granulomatous hepatitis in this case, as the illness developed shortly after self-treatment had started, and in due course resolved after it was stopped. Indomethacin had apparently been well tolerated over several years of regular use, and the nature of the hepatitis differed from that which has been reported in hepatotoxicity from indomethacin.

"The public should be made more aware of the potential for harmful effects from ingesting preparations of this sort, and doctors should become more alert to the possibility of their patients consuming these products without their knowlege.

S.C. Milazzo

The Queen Elizabeth Hospital
Woodville, S.A. 5011

CHAPTER SEVEN

A COURT ACTION

It is a matter of judgement in a court of law *when* Stuart McFarlane, his company or its servants learned of a link between the mussel and arthritis relief from the directors of Aquaculture Corporation, and whether they acted upon this knowledge.

That was to be settled in the New Zealand Supreme Court when McFarlane faced a $5 million law suit.

An item of vital interest to all concerned in the mussel/arthritis saga, was the publication in an American health magazine *'Bestways'* of a letter claiming the link was known and acted on *more than 10 years* before the parties facing each other in court, had met.

In its July 1980 issue, *'Bestways'* carried a letter from Mrs Arthur Eriksen, of Allen, in Texas, headed: 'Arthritis Medicine from the Sea — News of the Talented Discover'.

Mrs. Eriksen wrote:

Dear Bestways:

It was with great delight that we received a copy of your January 1980 edition.

The article by David Potterton entitled "Arthritis Medicine from the Sea" is a subject that is in my husband's heart, because he is the original researcher that discovered this miraculous cure in 1960. He has devoted his time, energy, and money — funding all of his own research — to this for twenty years. He is responsible for New Zealand being in the business of cultivating the green lipped mussel Perna canaliculus.

The first clinical evaluations covering the arthritis corrections were conducted by the Los Angeles College of Chiropractic in 1968. As a result of his efforts, in this, five out of five individuals responded favorably.

The next research was at the Autonomous University Medical School in Guadalajara, Mexico. Thirty-five people were selected on the basis of having suffered arthritis, without improvement for two years prior to the tests. This investigation resulted in 32 out of the 35 responding favorably.

With a dose rate of 12 capsules per day, 12 exhibited none of the symptoms they had had at the beginning of the 90-day period. Eleven had significant improvement and the balance were improved. Three did not finish the test for one reason or another.

Like all dedicated researchers, my husband was not interested in monetary returns, but why this substance did what it did. He pored over thousands of research papers in related fields and, as he is a recognized genius in instrumentation, systems control engineering, applied this expertise to the human body, the most superb of all systems. The thousands of sufferers of not only arthritis, but many more degenerative disorders, who have received relief with the mussel material is all the pay he needs.

I am interested in my husband's getting the recognition due him. I want him to be able to pass on the most important product of the past twenty years — his research. He has the keys to unlock the door of a new way of finding an answer not only to longer life, but a healthy vigorous longer life.

I would appreciate it if you could send me a copy of the January issue, as the person who brought the issue to us wanted Arthur's autograph on the magazine for the future because he believes that what Arthur has done is certainly worth one Nobel Award.

Sincerely,
Mrs. Arthur Eriksen,
Allen, TX.

On the same page the magazine carried 'An Answer from the Original Manufacturer of Perna canaliculus' —

Dear Bestways:

David Potterton, in his article "Arthritis Medicine from the Sea," has accurately described the development of sea farming of the New Zealand Mussel, Perna canaliculus, and confirmed its application as a natural source of health benefits.

The original manufacturer of the freeze-dried mussel powder, lyophilized homogenized mussel, is Aquaculture Corporation which began research on the nutritional *effects from sea mussels before 1967.*

Subsequent individual use and offshore tests have revealed the health benefits of the mineral and nutritional elements that are extracted from the sea and concentrated by the mussel as it feeds. As an elemental part of the food chain the mussel filters enormous quantities of water every day, efficiently converting the plankton and algae to high quality protein, complex carbohydrates, and unsaturated fats. Together with the natural balance of minerals and trace elements from the sea, it is not surprising that dramatic benefits have been noted in maintaining and restoring good health.

Mussels contain about the same amount of protein per ounce as beefsteak, but that's where the comparison stops; there is only a sixteenth of the fat and less than a quarter of the calories. Unlike steak, there is a high proportion of carbohydrates, about 20 percent of the dry mussel. This carbohydrate content is the source of mucopolysaccharides, which are known to be vital in human body chemistry. Only in the last few years, for instance, have bio-chemists discovered that mucopolysaccharides form an essential part of the wall of the human cell.

For further information, and for the encapsulated product of lyophilized homogenized mussel, called (trade-name), your readers may contact —

Aquaculture Corporation, 365 Convention Way, Redwood City, CA 94063

Sincerely,
R.W. Dorst, President.

Fascinated by this new developement I set out to find Mr. Eriksen. I had his telephone number, but called him for weeks in Allen, Texas, without success. I wrote to him hoping the address in the small town would be sufficient. A fortnight later he replied, from Plano, Texas:

December 15, 1982

The first freeze dried mussel nutriment extract product was produced in laboratory scale equipment fabricated, assembled and operated by me in the garage of my home in Mountainview, California in 1959, from the meats and body fluids of the specie mytilus Californianus, *known as the California Sea Mussel.*

The first arthritis correction was experienced by an

associate of mine at the Lockheed Missile and Space Division. He had been unable to grasp a pen to write his signature to documents. This was corrected in a matter of a week to two weeks without pain etc. The second person to achieve a correction was my 72-year old mother, who was riddled with rheumatic arthritis in every joint of her body, and was facing being a bed-ridden cripple for the rest of her life. In a matter of 30 days, she was well on her way to being completely free of arthritic symptoms. She continued to take the supplement daily, free of symptoms until her demise at the age of 79, due to an accident. She could do body push ups from the floor, and also Can-Can kickups, enjoying herself to the fullest.

In 1962, I formed the (trade-name) Company as a wholly owned proprietorship, using my Trademark (trade-name) to market the Supplement, also produced from the California Sea Mussel, making use of the commercial freeze drying facilities of Frank Oliver & Son at Watsonville, Calif. after the product had been certified to be fit for human consumption by the State of California Department of Health at Berkley, Calif.

In 1967 the (trade-name) Company was merged into Aquaculture Corporation, along with the transfer of all rights, knowhow, trademarks etc. Robert A. Gilmore and myself were the co-founders. Gilmore was elected President and myself as 1st Vice President, Orville H. Miller Treasurer, and Robert MacDonald as Secretary.

During 1967 a friend of mine who had been in the South East Pacific areas extensively, told me about a green mussel that was prevalent in that part of the world. I made inquiry of an import export food broker in San Francisco who located a commercial source from New Zealand (the green lipped mussel). I made arrangements to have 25 pounds of frozen meats to be delivered to San Francisco via Pan American Airways.

Upon its arrival I took a portion of it to Victor L. Loosanoff, the world's leading shell fish authority, for his examination and comment. Another portion was freeze-dried, using the facilities of Edward Hirschberg at South San Francisco, Calif.

Arrangements were subsequently made to obtain the green lipped mussel in a freeze dried state directly by air in 5 gal. tin containers.

Aquaculture Corporation was responsible for making arrangements with the Government of New Zealand to employ raft/rope suspension and hatchery techniques developed by

Dr. Loosanoff. The legal matters were conducted by Mr. Gilmore. The quality assurance provisions which I developed were handled by O.H. Miller, Ph.D. while I was involuntarily exiled from Aquaculture Corporation due to the personal harrassment and coercion of Aquaculture Corporation by the U.S. Food and Drug Administration. I served the Bechtel Group of Companies for two years on assignment in the Sahara Desert in Libya, North Africa, for their client, Occidental Petroleum Corporation, constructing and activating facilities totalling several hundred millions of dollars.

All marine species of mussels contain a full complement of nutriment. Nutriment is defined in dictionaries as 'something that nourishes or promotes growth and repairs the natural wastage of organic life'. Therefore nutriment can not only repair cell damage, but also promote the renewal of healthy cells and cell systems of all types. The use of mussel nutriment extracts accomplishes the correction, control and prevention of arthritic symptoms by replacing poorly functional cell systems of all types with properly functional cell systems. The interactions of these combined systems removes the symptoms of arthritis by correcting the basic causes of the disorders.

At this time I would like to emphasize that I have not received any profit from any of my activities over the intervening years, nor do I have any affiliation with any producer and/or marketer of the freeze dried mussel nutriment extracts originating in New Zealand or the Netherlands.

I am now retired from my domestic and foreign activities with the Bechtel Group Companies, having served them and their clients for a total of 23 years. I am a member of A.A.A.S and the New York Academy of Science.

* * *

Women's magazine readers in New Zealand were given some insight into Arthur Eriksen, when a firm manufacturing its own mussel extract in opposition to McFarlane's published a full-page advertisement about him. Headed: 'WILL THE REAL MUSSEL MIRACLE MAN PLEASE STEP FORWARD' it said:

'Many of the world's most exciting discoveries have been the byproduct of work on quite unrelated problems. One such accidental discovery is the now famous New Zealand green lipped mussel extract, known world-side as (here they used the product's trade-name).

'In 1954 instrumentation systems control engineer, Arthur Eriksen, was in the design phase of systems for a major power plant, when he ran across the problem of "fouling" by shellfish growing in the seawater intake tunnels. Such tunnels yielded a tremendous "harvest" of shellfish, mostly mussels. Could this "nuisance" be turned into a rich source of balanced nutrition, he thought?

'Using his own money, Eriksen embarked on a research program which led to shellfish cultivation and development facilities in Palo Alto, California. In this search for an economically viable product using the mussels, he developed a freeze-dried extract. Comprehensive laboratory testing showed the extract to be exceptionally suitable for human consumption.

'Now the real test, trial of the product by people. All the subjects who tried the extract found it quite acceptable to take and no reports of any discomfort were reported. But to Eriksen's surprise all reported positive benefits in their wellbeing, including improved joint movement, extra stamina and more energy. And so began an appreciation of the special nutritional properties which are exciting interest in (trade-name) around the world.

'In 1967 Eriksen resigned as Project Management Supervisor of a major corporation to found his own company for investigating the nutritional benefits of sea mussels, and directing field ecology survey programmes. In his research he discovered that the green lipped mussel, variety *Perna canaliculus,* found only in the unpolluted waters off the New Zealand coast, had many properties making it the most suitable for the freeze-drying extraction process.

'Shellfish were among the earliest inhabitants on Earth and fossil remains date the mussel back to the early Paleozoic Era. During the five hundred million years that it took for advanced life forms to evolve and colonise the land masses, the New Zealand green lipped mussel perfected a filter feeding system that is a true marvel of nature.

'Up to 10 gallons of seawater are filtered each day to obtain minerals and nutrients. The result is a shellfish containing a unique blend of amino-acids, chelated minerals, enzymes, mucopolysaccharides with traces of vitamins and other elements.

'While the mussel extract provides quite remarkable benefits, it is not a drug. It is a food, and (trade-name) is sold in health food shops around the world. It is non-toxic and apart from those naturally allergic to shellfish, can be taken on a continuing basis.

'The freeze-drying process produces a microbiologically stable extract, without damaging the important nutrients. Only the water is vaporized directly from frozen mussel, leaving moisture-free extract.

'The purity of the extract can only be guaranteed when it is produced from mussels, cultivated in carefully controlled marine farms, stresses Eriksen. The green lipped mussels used for (trade-name) grow on a matrix of ropes suspended in clear ocean currents off New Zealand's coastline. The water in these marine farms is strictly monitored daily for bacteriological, heavy metal or other pollution.

'After two years the mussels are harvested. Only after careful cleaning are the finest mussels chosen for producing the extract. Extensive analysis of the extract and careful quality control at every step ensures the guaranteed quality of (trade-name). While this process remains a trade secret, to (trade-name) users around the world, the benefits are well known.

'With the growing interest in (trade-name) comes a growing recognition of Arthur Eriksen, the true pioneer of the New Zealand green lipped mussel extract. This remarkable man developed and successfully marketed his first patent at 12 years age. He was granted a patent on extracting oil from vegetable material, using ion exchange, in 1952. He developed the control instumentation in data handling design of large scale space simulation facilities for the United States Air Force Systems Command and NASA. He also aided in the preparation of food for the NASA astronauts and much more. But perhaps he will become best known as the real "Mussel Miracle Man" — the man who gave New Zealand Green Lipped Mussel to the world.

* * *

When Arthur Eriksen produced his original product from the California sea mussel, he had 'no idea', he told me, that it had any therapeutic qualities.

"It was known to me that it had excellent nourishing qualities; but it was not until the testing phase of my pilot project — for toxicity and allergic responses — that I became aware of the potential therapeutic properties, including arthritis correction.

"All marine mussels possess arthritic therapeutic properties. Cultivated mussels, as they have been grown for hundreds of years in Holland, are preferred for their superior qualities, as opposed to wild mussels. The Holland mussel has superior nutrient and therapeutic properties, in some ways, to the New Zealand mussel, and vice versa.

"I ran across the New Zealand *Perna canaliculus* in my search for an inexpensive source of supply, and the Government of New Zealand sent some samples of this mussel to me... before McFarlane Laboratories was a thought in fisherman McFarlane's mind. It is a better mussel *only* from the standpoint of commercial utilization, i.e. rapid growth, higher meat to shell ratio, and higher total solids content."

After forming a company to make his product commercially available, Arthur Eriksen said he turned his mind to the questions: 'Why does such a little bit of this pure food do all these things? Why does it work?'

"I have," he said to me, "spent thousands of hours poring over thousands of research papers in fields such as physiology, biochemistry, nutritional biochemistry, animal husbandry, and medical research, and had many discissions with many leaders in these respective fields to unearth the clues. I did find 'why it works'; a 20-year study culminating in my treatise 'TOTAL NUTRIMENT THERAPY FOR ARTHRITIS', which contains an explanation for the mussel's ability to correct, control and prevent arthritis."

CHAPTER EIGHT

THE TESTIMONIALS

Within weeks of McFarlane Laboratories selling their capsules in pharmacies from Auckland to London, and Brisbane to Dublin, letters from arthritis sufferers began arriving at their offices.

Many requested additional information about the capsule and whether it could be harmful; many heard of it from other arthritics and wanted to know where it could be bought.

Ing. J.H. Moddemeijer, "El Ancladero", Apartado 8, Spain, wrote on 31 December 1979 —

'Thank you very much for your kind and helpful letter of 21 November last. In the meantime my wife went to Holland and succeeded to buy (trade-name) in Holland in a well known "Health Shop" there.

'To conclude this year I feel obliged to inform you about my miraculous experience with the ME. I told you already something about my background in my first letter of 1st November and that I badly suffered of chronic rheumatoid polyarthritis during the past months. From August on I have been treated here with all "hard medical drugs" of the pirarolones butaphenarolone, and corticosteroidgraeeps without any lasting result. Sometimes a certain relief but upon ceasing with a specific medicine after a few days from bad to worse again. My whole condition became gradually worse. I felt poisoned by medicines, lost my appetite and felt depressed. We wonder, as I saw the wheel chair coming towards me. I stopped therefore all cures and felt a little better when the side effects disappeared. At that time the balance was:

'Active arthritis in the right knee accompanied by a serious bursitis, active arthritis in right ankle joints, right thumb and indicator finger, left wrist with crippled 4 fingers, right shoulder and shoulder blade and also some pain in adjoining ribs.

'On 13th December I started with (trade-name). The first 8 days no change. On the ninth day increasing pain in all affected joints with slight fever till the 13th day (without fever and decreasing pain). On the 14th day all other joints which were affected in the preceding years showed symptoms of becoming active again accompanied by again slight fever. On the 15th day, however, I awoke for the first time with hardly any arthritic pain, although stiffness and immobility still remained. From the 16th to the 20th everything improved gradually which caused a feeling of well-being. From the 21st to 23rd day another revival of arthritic pain and slight fever but now in all joints affected now and his former years. But on the 24th day this all gone. From there on a gradual decrease of muscle tensions, stiffness and a slowly increasing mobility in all affected joints. Swollen right knee and ankle slowly diminishing. On 32nd day able to walk again. On 42nd day mobility, apart from some trouble of joint deformations, nearly normal for any age and now on the last day of this year (the 48th day) hardly any pain, pleasant mobility.

'Mobility in all joints affected now and in former years. Swolleness in right knee and ankle decreased fairly rapidly. Remarkably I noticed also a regressing tendency in deformations of joints, tendons, etc even in those of earlier date with which I had already leaned to live with. My present condition can be resumed as follows:

'I am able to use all affected joints again without pain and with only some slight limitations and I can now carry out again the usual odd jobs around the house. I can walk again without trouble although I still have to be careful with the use of my right leg as both knee and ankle joints were rather badly damaged.

'Six weeks ago I had to pass my days as a still dynamic person in bed or on a couch. A sad prospect! I also noticed a beneficial side effect. Small cuts and skin grazes are now healing, as I estimate, about twice as quickly as before. My story would not be complete if I did not mention someting of my amnesis.

'Heretary *(sic)* arthritis can be excluded as this disease does not occur among my ancestors and relatives. During the late world war I was a P.O.W. in Japanese prison-camps in S.E. Asia. Apart from the usual tropical diseases, I suffered in the camps from a severe avitaminosis leading to a nearly complete paralysis of my digestive system (principally because of lack of vitamin B). After the war it restored itself but never reached a state of full reconvalescence. The system showed weak spots especially in the bowels. It never caused serious trouble as I learned to avoid some kinds of food and I stopped taking alcohol. I realised that my metabolism and assimilation were not 100% and that when arthritis manifested itself about 10 years ago the cause could be some defect in the most complex part of metabolism and assimilation, being that of proteins and compositions such as hormones. It is for this reason that M.E. appealed to me so much. Fortunately my blood pressure is still perfect. My blood analysis is generally very satisfactory, except a too high percentage of reactive protein... I told my Spanish rheumatologist frankly about my successful trial with (trade-name). He was amazed. Had heard something of M.E. from his colleagues. But only rumours as (trade-name) is not available in Spain to test it. I showed him the way to order it by mail in England.

'Thanking you from the bottom of my heart for the development of your harmless and most beneficial medicine.'

Mrs. I. Vernon, who worked in a medical practice at Berrima, NSW 2577, wrote on 6 July 1982:

'I have suffered from osteo-arthritis for years and it has given me considerable pain, particularly in my fingers and latterly my feet.

'As I have worked for doctors for some years, and presently am employed by an excellent G.P. in Moss Vale, I received very good care, but there was a limit to the types of anti-inflammatory drugs they could prescribe, and each one caused symptoms making it impossible to continue treatment.

'I commenced taking the 230 m.g. capsules of (trade-name), and within about a fortnight, to my amazement I was suddenly aware that I did not have the pain I had become so accustomed to. I felt better in so many ways, I suppose because the pain had lessened so considerably, however, my general health seems to have improved.

'I am now on my fourth bottle of (trade-name) and intend to continue with (it) for the rest of my life if necessary. I told my doctor, who was delighted, and his wife, who is the local pharmacist, stocks it now.

'Although my fingers will always remain deformed, the swelling is still reducing.

'Thank you most sincerely for the help I have received, the relief from pain which I thought I would just have to put up with. I am 54 years old, but not ready yet to sit in a chair and forego all the things I wish to do.'

Then — four months later — she reported:

'Even the bony nodules on the joints in some of my fingers have reduced in size, and presently I am taking only two of the 230 mg. capsules per day, (I increase this to three per day if I feel pain, and this occurs mostly when I have had a large amount of typing to do).

'There was a period of time (approximately three weeks) when I had run out of the capsules, and was unable to get any. I became quite concerned, as the pain returned (about a week after running out of the capsules) and with a "vengeance". I felt ill with pain and stiffness in my hands, feet and neck, however I have since found a supplier, and now keep a stock of about three bottles at all times. I did feel that the condition exacerbated, although this may have been a psychological matter, however I am a fairly practical person and feel that my arthritis really did worsen. I omitted to mention that I am able to grip with much more strength, as I had lost a lot of strength in my hands.'

* * *

On 19 July 1977, Mrs. Marjorie N. Dwyer of St. Kilda, Melbourne, wrote to the mussel extract company —

'I am writing to inform you the beneficial result obtained from one (1) bottle of (trade-name) (125 caps.).

'My left arm was powerless, and I could not walk properly, only shuffle along. Over the past four years my arthritis grew progressively worse and I was in constant pain.

'I took the prescribed dose of five capsules a day, and approximately the 10th day the pain become almost unbearable and was intense for three to four days.

'Since then, the (to me) miracle has occurred. My left arm is restored to former use, I can carry and lift easily, I am walking freely and, which is more wonderful, the pain has disappeared completely for the first time in many years. I have a feeling of well being and an eagerness for work, and am becoming very active and mobile. I am telling as many people I come in contact with who suffer similar complaints.

'Please accept my heartfelt thanks and all good wishes."

Five years later I asked her to describe her present condition. She wrote to me:

'Every now and again, say five/six months, after I've been

running around busier than usual, some twinges start up the shins — which area was particularly sore to the point of infected arthritis and bed rest with feet up. So when (I get) a twinge I go back to (trade-name), five a day with meals for a week — and the pains disappear. This "booster" treatment is all I need to control the arthritis all over my body — thankfully"

***

On 29 September 1982, Mrs. Joan C. Johnson of Sherwood, Nottingham, in England, wrote to the manufacturing company:

'I only wish (trade-name) had been available 30 years ago when I first started with rheumatoid arthritis, because I feel certain I would not have developed the deformities I now have. Since taking (trade-name) all stiffness and inflammation have left me... I cannot walk very far at one time because my feet and ankles become extremely painful, they are very deformed as are my hands. Besides having rheumatoid I have a gastric ulcer which has not troubled me at all since taking (trade-name). I can eat anything without any discomfort.'

Mrs. Johnson said in a letter to me two months later:

'Since taking (trade-name) my rheumatoid arthritis has remained quiescent and I feel certain that if it were not for the painful deformities I developed prior to taking (trade-name) I would be unaware of having the disease. About two weeks after I started taking (trade-name) I felt absolutely dreadful; my condition worsened, but that passed and I began to get better and have never looked back. Quite possibly this initial setback puts people off and they stop taking (trade-name), but I must stress that this feeling passes and to be fairly judged (trade-name) should be taken for six months non-stop at the maximum daily dosage.

'May I add that, besides looking after myself, my home and the garden, as well as working full time, until last Christmas I had to look after my elderly husband who has Parkinsons Disease, Dementia and is incontinent. My doctor says she does not know how I managed, because I am very noticeably disabled in my hands, feet and knees (one knee being an artificial replacement) but I can quite truthfully say that I do not think I could have done it if I had not been taking (trade-name).'

***

Mr. Ron Gundesen of Mangakino, New Zealand, wrote to

the company on 21 June 1982—

'Four years ago I started running on the road in road races and marathons, developing arthritis in the process. A number of doctors and specialists I visited claimed that all I could do was forget the running, as the arthritis was that bad nothing could be done. All their anti-inflammatory medication was of no success. I then turned to the green lipped mussel and after 2½ bottles of capsules I could feel a change in my joints. I have now taken 31 bottles of capsules which has resulted in me running 15 marathons and numerous varied distance races. I completed three marathons in the space of 36 days.'

Five months later he reported to me, amplifying his earlier letter:

'I started running after a lapse of 15 years and sustained pains in joints and muscles which I firstly and naturally put down to age and the sudden commencement of running. My aches worsened and I sought medical advice and got all sorts of results until finally I was x-rayed. The results were demoralising. Every bit of advice as, "you have had it. Give running away, you have arthritis and if you keep running you will suffer and do (yourself) damage..."

'I have now completed in two overseas Internationals in England and Japan. The capsules... got me running free of pain and suffering, and that is all I want out of life. At no time have I had a re-occurence of the arthritis since the commencement of the mussel. I have taken 36 bottles to date.'

Mrs. Thelma Pitt-Turner of Palmerston North, wrote:

'I have suffered with arthritis for many years and have had rheumatic specialists' attention. They have advised me in the past that there was nothing they could do for me.

'About five years ago I commenced jogging and over the last couple of years have become a registered harrier. I am New Zealand's oldest registered road runner and have won two National Titles, third place in a Provincial and in 1981 was placed third in the World Veteran Road Race Championships, 10 km., beating USA and Western Germany. I have also participated in half marathons (13 miles).

'I believe that (trade-name) has benefited me by strengthening my muscles as well as increasing my staying power. I have had no recurrence of arthritis. People, as well as medical practitioners, are amazed at my capabilites of my running at the age of 79.

A nursing sister from a Catholic hospital in Cork wrote to the company on 18 December 1978:

'Thank you very much for your kind letter and much appreciated information re Mussel Extract. I should have answered your letter long ago but I waited to see how the treatment affected me personally.

'Now I am very pleased to tell you my condition has improved very noticeably especially in my cervical spine and in my knees. As I already told you I have rheumatoid arthritis in my dorsal and lumbar spine also, but in August I had a few treatments of deep heat and massage on those regions and as yet I am not sure what effect the Mussel Extract has had on those parts. In time I will know, but I am presently very well and able to do a full day's work thank God.

'I have got many friends of mine interested in the product and it is wonderful to be able to say to them "It's not a drug". With drugs one is always very cautious and we so often see the side effects in our nursing experience. I have tried giving them to some of the old people here but somehow they expect an instant cure and of course that can't happen.

'I have taken three courses — five x 230 mg. every day for 22 days and I will continue for some time I hope. Quite obviously the longer one is suffering from arthritis — the longer one has to take Mussel Extract.

'I am glad you are coming to Dublin in March and I look forward to meeting you. In the meantime have a good rest and enjoy a happy and holy Christmas with many blessing in 1979.

'God bless you.

What was her condition three years later?

'I am very happy to tell you that (trade-name) or mussel extract has done a great job for me and is still proving to be the magic mussel. As you have learned from the files in McFarlane's Lab I have taken this treatment for some years now, and thank God I am still enjoying wonderful relief from arthritis. For the first two years I took the capsules more or less daily and as the symptoms lessened I reduced my intake to one bottle (110 capsules) every month. This summer I was able to do without any capsules for six months so you see how well I have been...

'I feel that (trade-name) has been a great breakthrough and

no other treatment is as safe and effective or simple; for one thing it is *not* a drug and there are no side-effects... Many people I know have used it with good results, but there are many also who have taken it and found no relief whatever.'

CHAPTER NINE

THE GUINEA PIGS

'Where angels fear to tread...' a newspaperman will blithely march. Uninhibited by scientific parameters involving double-blind crossover trials and the fine measurement of pain, a reporter will arbitrarily select a reader with a disease, hand over the claimed 'cure' and await the results — assuming they come before the story loses its impact.

So it was with two newspapers on opposite sides of the Atlantic, whose reports put the New Zealand crude mussel extract on 'trial'.

'Trial' No. 1 took place in a column written by Mr. Dennis Laxton. He told his Reading, Berks., readers:

"The misery of arthritis is torturing more people, young and old, every year. Although research into the cause and cure of this crippling disease is going on all over the world, nobody has yet come up with a satisfactory remedy.

"But I am impressed by the claims of Mr. John Croft, a British-born and trained scientist now based in New Zealand, who is working on a unique form of treatment.

"He told me about it while he was over here visiting his laboratory's U.K. headquarters in Reading. Briefly, it's an extract from the New Zealand green-lipped mussel *(Perna canaliculus)*, a shellfish found only in the unpolluted waters around those shores.

"After five years of trials, it is now being marketed in several countries, including Britain. And Mr. Croft states that doctors have reported 'at least 60 per cent success rate treating rheumatoid arthritis'. He also says that many of the patients were chronic cases who had not responded to other forms of treatment.

"Having seen the deformed, claw-like hands of so many sufferers, watched them trying to creep around, gasping with pain, and heard their stories of sleepless nights, I thought Mr. Croft's discovery deserved serious consideration.

"Now, a 69-year-old Caversham housewife, a victim of severe arthritis for the last six years, has agreed to try the capsules — with the approval of her doctor. She will take the prescribed five a day for a month, all the time usually needed for a definite improvement in most patients.

"Mr. Croft, wisely, does not guarantee improvement 'because people react differently to the same treatments and I believe that no one treatment for arthritis will suit everyone.' But I'll be charting Mrs. A's progress week by week.

"I don't intend to publish the trade name of the product unless there are positive results at the end of the course. And I hope readers will take my word for it that the only personal gain I shall get from this experiment is the satisfaction of seeing this lady happy again."

At the end of week one of his 'arthritic experiment' Laxton reported that 'Mrs. A' was still limping. "She says she's had slightly more pain than usual in the past few days. But that, I explained to the 69-year-old Caversham housewife, is good news. It's a common experience for many people who have gained lasting relief after taking a full course of the extract... Apparently it's like the lager which reaches places that others don't and flushes out the cause of the trouble.

"I also learned this week." said Laxton, "that there is evidence that the relief can't be credited to 'mind over matter'.. Dogs and cats, often victims of arthritis in old age, have been successfully treated with the same capsules. And there is no way an animal can be 'conned' into believing a remedy will work to such an extent that there is a psychologically-induced cure."

Week three found 'Mrs. A' still limping. "That's how I started off last week, and it doesn't sound like progress," wrote the columnist. "But she says she has had one pain-free day, a rare event in the six years she has been crippled in the right hip and knee by the disease... one day, after only three weeks' treatment, is at least hopeful. She celebrates her 70th birthday next Wednesday and I'm hoping she gets a gift from *Perna canaliculus* — to use the mussel's posh name."

By week four's end 'Mrs. A' had found no lasting improvement, but the one day free of pain she experienced half-way through the course of treatment had encouraged her to continue.

On week six a jubilant Laxton wrote: "It's literally all systems go for a successful conclusion eventually. My capsule-taker is experiencing everything predicted by British-born scientist, John Croft, now working in New Zealand on a new treatment for the crippling disease.

"She is taking five capsules a day, containing an extract from the New Zealand green-lipped mussel.

Doctors who have tested the remedy, confirm a 60 per cent success rate in cases of rheumatoid arthritis, and between 30 and 50 per cent for osteoarthritis.

'Mrs. A' just turned 70, had been a victim of osteo-arthritis — the worst of the two, and the most difficult to treat — for six years. If her condition doesn't improve, she will have to have an operation on her right hip.

During the fourth week of the course, she had a complete day free of pain, for the first time in all those years.

Last week, for the one day, the pain was severe.

I checked this with Mr. Croft in New Zealand, and his telex reply was: 'It's beginning to take effect strongly.'

Apparently, many patients experience a temporary increase of pain in the affected joints at this stage, which means, without going into the medical details, that the cause of the trouble is being flushed out."

Then week seven — *'The Breakthrough'*.

"Mrs. A', wrote Laxton, "is experiencing successive pain-free nights for the first time since the crippling disease struck here six years ago... a couple of days ago 'Mrs. A' told me: 'the pain used to wake me up in the middle of the night, and I stayed awake. It was something I learned to put up with, but I've slept soundly every night for the past week.

'For years I've had great difficulty in getting out of bed in the morning and going downstairs. The only way I could get down was by leaning heavily on the banister rail and taking it slowly, step by step. During the past week, I've been able to walk down, just holding the rail. It's wonderful.'"

Laxton promised:

"If the improvement in her condition is maintained I'll identify the product, and tell you about it next month."

He did.

"The condition in her hip is definitely improved. Now she's experiencing the same reaction in her right knee. She is still taking the capsules, but considering the lady's age and the fact that she has osteoarthritis, it may well be several more months before I know the outcome."

He published the name of the product.

"We made this decision because arthritis is becoming a scourge. If anything can be done to relieve it, even slightly, we have helped somebody."

* * *

In Florida, USA, in April 1981, *The Sun* newspaper selected a group of arthritics for an experiment the paper called *'Break Through'*. The purpose of the plan was *'to prove or disprove that the extract of the green-lipped mussel of New Zealand could bring relief from the misery and pain of arthritis, a disease so prevalent among our senior citizens.'*

Fifty-one sufferers were chosen, with a common goal: to find whether the mussel worked or it didn't.

On 3 September 1981, after five months taking the capsules supplied by a health and diet-aids company, the guinea-pigs reported back to the newspaper. *The Sun's* bannerhead line said: 'ARTHRITIS EXPERIMENT PROVES A SUCCESS' and beneath it, Ned F. Kailing wrote:

"Plan *Break Through* is a success. We have exceeded our expectations and can now point to a 70% positive reaction. It is possible that this percentage will increase before we terminate the plan. We are into our fifth month and it is intensely gratifying to see our skepticism disappear with the enthusiastic results proclaimed by those participating in the plan. We have learned much from plan *Break Through*, of greatest importance is the fact that the green-lipped mussel does have a therapeutic value for many of those afflicted with arthritis. I am not convinced," said Kailing, "that it is a panacea for all arthritics or that it brings an ultimate cure. But! What I have seen thus far is unequivocal proof that we are better off for having this natural food supplement (hi-vitamin, mineral concentrate) than not to have it. As mentioned, I was a doubting Thomas. I have osteoarthritis in the lower lumbar region of my spine. My wife has rheumatoid arthritis in her hands. Yes: we have improved considerably. Those who are participating in the plan will tell you of their results — some have been startling..."

On another page *The Sun* told the background story of the guinea-pig experiment.

It said:

"At first, 69-year-old Walter Shakotko was pessimistic.

He was convinced nothing -- not even the green tablets with a fishy smell -- could relieve the constant pain he had endured from many years of arthritis.

Shakotko lives in Kings Point, where he frequently performs odd jobs for his neighbours. He enjoys working with his hands. But his swollen knuckles and joints, characteristic of some forms of arthritis, made this virtually impossible.

'I couldn't shake hands; I couldn't hold a tool; I couldn't grab a cup of coffee,' he explained.

Through the years Shakotko had tried the gamut of prescribed remedies, aspirin and other pain relievers. But, 'nothing helped.'

Many of Shakotko's neighbours — also arthritics — were convinced that the green tablets they were taking as part of a layman's experiment brought them relief from arthritis.

The pills contain an extract from the green-lipped mussel, native to New Zealand waters.

The pills are manufactured in the United States under the name of (trade-name) by the American Diet-aids company, based in Orangeburg, N.Y.

Recently, claims have been made that the food supplement could relieve the symptoms of arthritis.

Ned Kailing, and arthritic for many years, found relief from (trade-name).

Kailing, a retired businessman living in Kings Point, decided to spearhead an experiment to test the pills.

'We have arthritic people here by the dozens,' Kailing said. Kings Point and nearby Sun City Center are major retirement communities in south Hillsborough Country.

After noting a decrease in pain in his back after taking (trade-name), Kailing last April organized about 50 residents of Kings Point and Sun City Center to begin taking daily doses of the pills and chart the results.

American Dietaids agreed to supply Kailing with enough (trade-name) to carry out his program.

After spending several sleepless nights because of excessive pain, Shakotko agreed to join in Kailing's experiment. Although he agreed to take the tablets four times a day, he didn't put much faith in them.

'I tried everything else. This was just another crack-pot thing,' he said.

But after the first week of treatment, Shakotko began to

notice changes. He continued the regimen.

Today, after more than two months, Shokotko is a believer.

'Look what I'm doing,' he said, flexing his hand. 'These knuckles were so sore, I couldn't touch them. Today I can shake hands and squeeze the knuckles.

'It's a miracle to me, and it's not in my head. In my estimation this has done it,' Shakotko said, twisting a bottle of (trade-name) in his hand. 'I've never gotten relief such as this.'

While Kailing claims more than a 70 per cent success rate among participants in his program, others question its effects on arthritis.

Much of the skepticism centres on the fact that the product has not been scientifically tested on arthritics.

The Arthritis Foundation warned arthritics about the 'unproven' product.

'The reason we do not condone or endorse the product is because there is no scientific evidence that proves what it claims to do,' said Floyd Pennington, vice president for education for the Arthritis Foundation's national office in Atlanta. 'It may indeed provide temporary relief... but we would not suggest it. We don't have scientific evidence to support it.'

The lack of test data prompted the Food and Drug Administration last year to ban the import of the key ingredient in (trade-name) — the mussel extract — into the United States. The ban will diminish supplies of (trade-name).

The controversy began when a New Zealand author, John Croft, toured the United States promoting his book which claimed that the extract could relieve arthritis symptoms.

The book was promoted along with the (trade-name) tablets, and the FDA stepped in.

The product was classified as an 'unapproved drug' because health claims were made about it, said William Grigg, director of press relations for the FDA.

The ban was implemented because no scientific laboratory tests were conducted to substantiate the claims that the extract had an effect on arthritis.

According to FDA officials, the company distributing or manufacturing the product is responsible for conducting the scientific tests.

But American Dietaids, which manufactures (trade-name) and distributes it in the United States, says it will not fight the ban or conduct the tests.

The FDA 'is a difficult agency to go through. There is very little we can do to get them to lift the ban,' said Reynald Swift, vice president of marketing for American Dietaids.

Fighting the FDA would require a 'huge investment', Swift said. 'We've adoped a wait-and-see attitude.'

Swift said the (trade-name) stock is almost out, but the company plans to keep Kailing's experiment supplied with (trade-name) as long as it can.

Kailing says his personal experience has made him a staunch believer.

A few years ago, a physician told Kailing the arthritis in his back would get progressively worse and he'd probably be restricted to a wheelchair.

'I tried everything I could get my hands on to relieve the pain,' said the 72-year-old Kings Point resident.

Kailing's wife, Dorothy, 74, also suffered from arthritis. She had lost 50 per cent of the mobility in her hands. Flexing them was almost impossible.

After the couple learned of the product from Croft's book, they began taking it.

The Kailings soon noticed results. Dorothy could easily stretch and flex her hands with no pain. Ned could turn his upper body with little pain.

Then Kailing got an idea for the experiment.

Originally the project began with 35 participants. American Dietaids agreed to supply Kailing with tablets free of charge.

Interest in the project spread through the community and the number of participants swelled to 65.

'How do you turn down people when they cry when you interview them? They beg you. It's pretty hard to say no,' Kailing said.

People who endure the pain of arthritis 'grasp at straws', he explained. 'That's what our people are doing here. After being in pain for years, you'll try anything.'

Kailing hopes his test results will persuade officials to lift the ban.

But according to the FDA and the Arthritis Foundation, Kailing's project is worthless because it relies on testimonial evidence. When participants in the program periodically visit Kailing, he charts how they are feeling. No doctor is overseeing the program.

'By not being a doctor, (Kailing) is not qualified to carry out the study,' said Martin Katz, compliance officer for the FDA district office in Orlando. 'He's relying on testimonial research, which is the worst kind. It's not controlled.'

The lack of medical supervision makes it almost impossible to determine if a participant's relief is real, Katz said.

Katz would have a hard time convincing 78-year-old Irene Hanck, who says (trade-name) diminished pain and swelling in her hands.

If the availability of (trade-name) is cut off, 'I'd be furious,' she said.

Hanck's sentiments are felt by many who found relief in (trade-name) through Kailing's experiment.

After taking daily doses of (trade-name) 76-year-old Ruth Godfrey was able to return to hobbies she had abandoned because of pain and deformities in her hands from arthritis.

"I can't write too well and it was hard for me to sew or knit." said Godfrey. "My hands were so bad I couldn't hold a pen."

Arthritis medication and aspirin were prescribed by a physician, but Godfrey said she couldn't tolerate them. She turned to the mussel extract.

Within five or six weeks, Godfrey was able to close her hands and make a fist.

'I'm knitting and I'm sewing and I'm trying to write." she said.

Godfrey doesn't think the FDA ban is necessary.

"They ban things and test them for so long, by the time you can get it, you're too far gone."

For about eight years, Jeannette Hagan, 70, endured the constant throbbing of arthritis in her fingers. After taking (trade-name) for six weeks, she said her fingers no longer throbbed and the swelling lessened.

Hagan had always refused to take arthritis medication, even aspirin. "I don't believe in medicine, but I don't consider this a medicine," she said of (trade-name) tablets. "This is a health food."

But medical officials say the experiment participants may be misinterpreting their decrease in pain. One characteristic of arthritis, doctors say, is that symptoms often disappear and reappear later. These disappearances are called remissions.

Those in Kailing's program who claim (trade-name) has diminished their symptoms may be experiencing remission, said Dolores Homb, director of the Arthritis Foundation's Gulf Coast Branch.

The danger is that arthritis may abandon proven medical treatment and replace it with unproven treatments such as (trade-name) Homb said.

But Kailing believes the effects are real and that the people who claim the tablets help them will be able to create enough public pressure to change the FDA ban.

"The FDA is viewing this as a drug. It's not a cure for arthritis — it's a relief," Kailing said.

CHAPTER TEN

ACTIVE INGREDIENT?

Paul Gregory, 40, was a Senior Lecturer in Biochemistry at the Royal Melbourne Institute of Technology when he became involved in an investigation of the New Zealand green-lipped mussel. He is a B.Sc.(Hons.), M.Sc.(Dist.), (Lon.) and was, at the time, a member of the RMIT Council.

The Institute has staff specialising in immunology, pathology, haematology, biochemistry, microbiology and physiology and is the largest institute of its kind in the Southern Hemisphere. It has 28,500 students.

It was over dinner in Melbourne that Paul Gregory first heard of the mussel and claims about its efficacy in the treatment of arthritis. Jim Broadbent, who heads the marketing company handling (trade-name) in Australia and several overseas countries was expanding on the mussel's anti-inflammatory role. Broadbent said the problem that faced McFarlane Laboratories was that they could not fractionate the mussel extract and find its active ingredient or ingredients.

Gregory, olive-skinned, moustachioed and with a blunt manner, recalls the conversation. "Jim said that John Croft, the company's marine biologist in Auckland, thought its efficacy might involve an integral balance of minerals, to which I replied, *'Bullshit!'*".

He'd had another sip of Broadbent's good claret and had gone on: "If it (the active ingredient) is there, it can be fractionated. If it can survive the gastro-intestinal tract and be absorbed; if it can go through all the growing, the harvesting, the processing, the pelletising, the encapsulation, the storage and then *still* survive what happens to it in the gut — it's obviously stable and able to be isolated."

Broadbent, an enthusiast and ideas-man with as forthright a manner as his dinner-guest said: "OK. If you think you're so good why don't you give it a try?"

"I replied," said Gregory, "that I was teaching full time. That I was a biochemist involved in consultative industrial chemistry and that I was very busy. However, maybe there were a couple of RMIT students interested in studying for their masters' degrees who could be interested. Jim asked me what that would cost. I said I felt such an investigation of the mussel would make a superb literature study for a couple of masters' students to let them try and get their teeth around; and to see what they came up with in the laboratory, given the controversial press associated with the product." He then named to Broadbent a figure covering each student for a two-year investigation.

It wasn't long before an arrangement between RMIT and McFarlanes was reached. Paul Gregory explained to me his attitude to the investigation. "I'd heard all about the Gibsons' work in Glasgow; I'd read the experts who said the work was all right and those who said it wasn't. Over in Auckland Dr. Tom Miller was doing work on the mussel, using rats, and we thought we might co-operate. He was working on an aqueous fraction of water soluble compounds and he suggested that maybe I should work on the lipid (fats and fatlike materials that are generally insoluble in water, but are soluble in common organic solvents) fraction and see if in fact there were any steroid-type, anti-inflammatory compounds or prostaglandins in it." (Prostaglandins are derived from unsaturated fatty acids and are involved in inflammation. Drugs like aspirin and indomethacin inhibit the formation of prostaglandins.)

"There had never been an extensive analysis done of the mussel; there were only indications that there were certain fatty acids and that there was a presence or absence of various other compounds... so there was a likelihood of several ingredients being there that nobody knew about. They'd done nothing on small, soluble molecules such as aspirin; or water-soluble anti-inflammatory compounds. So it was wide open." The RMIT and McFarlanes came to a firm agreement similar to research collaboration between drug companies and research centres all over the world, and the two masters degree students began work on the mussel meat, and in its brown, freeze-dried form. "The two students set about their task with enthusiasm and soon we started to see some results. They broke it down to identify which of its compounds were water-soluble and which were soluble in organic solvents.

"They found the lipid-soluble fraction had no anti-inflammatory activity whatsoever. So it seemed the whole area in which the project was to proceed was almost closed off at Day One! It meant that if the project was going to survive, we had to switch to the other area that Dr. Miller was working on — the aqueous fraction.

"In addition to trying to identify, isolate and purify the active component, we also had a number of other tasks to perform. We had to determine:—

1. Whether the anti-inflammatory model was effective (i.e. whether it exhibited false positives or false negatives and if so to make the necessary adjustments.)
2. We would want to know whether the compound could prevent inflammation if it was administered before the inflammatory agent. In other words if it acted *prophylactically,* or
3. To determine the effect of administering the compound after inflammation had occurred to determine whether there was a *therapeutic* effect.

"These tasks in fact were the basis of one student's project. The importance of controlling the experiment against false positive results could perhaps be better explained using the following analogy. Suppose we wanted to test whether a compound was effective against a bee sting. If the animal didn't get stung at all then one could assume that since there was no inflammation that the compound adminstered was 100% effective. This is a false positive and if included in a set of results causes serious errors in the subsequent statistical analysis. In the same manner one must be sure that strong inflammatory response is observed before administering the anti-inflammatory compound."

Gregory and his students had spent the specified two years probing the mussel in the laboratory. After the first six months had been spent 'chasing false trails' and getting the experiments started, a decision was made to look first at the small molecules, 'because most of the known anti-inflammatory drugs are small molecules'.

"But to our surprise," said Gregory, "there was no activity. It wasn't the molecule the size of aspirin or indomethacin (the basis of the well-known anti-inflammatory swallowed by millions of arthritics — Indocid); nor was it the size of penicillamine, gold or copper. We worked our way through, and to our surprise it was the *largest* group of molecules that had the anti-inflammatory activity in it. By virtue of the spectroscopic properties it cannot be a nucleic acid — DNA or RNA — and therefore it appeared to be a protein." (Proteins are highly complex nitrogenous compounds found in all animal and vegetable tissues and are essential for the growth and repair of the body.) "It was graded at a molecular weight of greater than 5,000.

"We then had to fractionate that fraction into its component molecules, to determine if it was one or more molecules that actually had the activity. We've had a couple of 'hiccups' because we've had difficulty in staining the protein (for identification in experiments). We are using an isoelectric focussing technique because most of these molecules have charges, positive and negative. The charge distribution for various proteins varies; in a given set of conditions they carry different proportions of positives and negatives. Therefore, when you put them across an electrical potential, the negatively-charged ones will move to the positive terminal; and they will move at different rates. In the isoelectric focussing process you see a banding and you can separate them.

"We have now managed to fractionate this big active protein fraction and subdivide it into approximately 15 bands. There is still work to be done to determine if each of these bands is homogenous" (uniform in structure) "but that can be done with other means.

"At the moment we are going through (this was in early 1983) a very slow, methodical process during which you just can't cut corners. We have been able to separate the bands in a qualitative scale, now we are moving towards a quantitative process. At the moment we have to repeat the small scale purification over and over until we've gathered enough to test each fraction on a rat model."

In tests on rat footpads made to swell deliberately by the introduction of a foreign agent, ultra-sensitive instruments are needed to gauge the degree of swelling and the degree of its reduction. Inflammation is generated chemically to imitate inflammation caused by arthritis in humans. The sea-weed extract — carrageen — which is used to provoke this reaction, is a polysaccharide, and its sugar composition makes it similar to the cell walls of bacteria, which cause an antigenic response in the body when they invade. "Immediately you inject it," explains Gregory, "bits of it break off and the body's immune cells tend to migrate to where it is, the same way they migrate to where the bacteria get in, and they elicit this response which then causes inflammation."

It will be on a rat paw that experiments will be conducted to determine which of the 15 fractions has the vital activity which could change arthritics' lives...

"We will have by then purified it 1,000 times from the volume of crude mussel extract we have extracted it from. That means only 1,000th part of the average gelatin-encapsulated mussel extract has activity: the rest is useless."

And where will this lead?

Paul Gregory will not be persuaded to dream dreams. He is a scientist. He only believes in facts he or his colleagues have established, and then only after they have been established over and over again. He is interested only in having a molecule he can 'accurately describe', knowing its precise isoelectric point, its protein characteristics, its associated compounds, its lipid group, its glyco group, its gross composition, its molecular sequence, whether or not it contains a rare amino-acid. And "whether or not it has a molecule such as aspirin — *dare I say it?* — incorporated into it. Because it seems a fairly powerful sort of molecule."

Then — with his industrial chemist's 'hat on' he says: "I will hopefully patent it. What I will be patenting is a molecule which has anti-inflammatory properties, which nobody else has. A new anti-inflammatory protein! It will then need somebody to work on a way of preparing it commercially, to extract it in bulk. We have to produce enough of the active material and then we must try it out. The pure material should be tried first by injection, then orally, with a 'label' of some sort so we can detect if it is in fact getting across the gut and into the bloodstream."

And if it isn't absorbed?

"Well it means that it's nothing more than a placebo. As a scientist I am determined that if this is the situation it has to be demonstrated."

And if it is demonstrated that it actually crosses the gut and gets into the bloodstream?

Gregory says simply: "If somebody comes up with an anti-inflammatory drug that has none of the side effects that present anti-inflammatory drugs have, they will effectively collar the world market. Total world sales of anti-inflammatory drugs at the moment amount to about $1,200 million a year, most of them taken by people who have rheumatism or some form of arthritis."

McFarlanes and the RMIT have signed a joint patent agreement, with the patent *rights* going to McFarlanes. "Then presumably when the money starts coming in they will start shovelling funds into RMIT for further research. So we will get the research money and the kudos for having isolated the active ingredient, which I am not suggesting at this moment, is a cure for arthritis.

"When I started on this I was cynical. It was just another project my students and I were working on. But when we showed we could fractionate and were getting closer, of course I became excited. But I was getting into an area in which I wasn't really competent. As soon as we started getting into mechanics and started to vie with the inflammatory experts around the world, I began to think: *'Hell's teeth!* Why don't I know more about this area so I can chase it?'"

His work threw him into a no-man's land between, on the one hand arthritics who had claimed the mussel had rid them of their aches and pains, and on the other, the medical Establishment and its intolerance of 'quack' remedies and fringe-medical claims. "Because I am a scientist I lean towards the medicos. I am still not convinced, through any scientific fact, that (trade-name) works on humans.

"The Gibsons' work, when you examine it, and look at the

statistics of it, is found wanting. So is Huskisson's work" (at St. Bartholemew's Hospital, London).

"The real problem with many trials is that the dosages worked out by John Croft were quite arbitrary. They had no relationship with the milligrams-per-kilos-of-weight associated with the animal tests. Statistics arrived at by the Gibsons were not powerful enough; the work was not adequately controlled.

"But having said all that — there is no doubt there *is* some anti-inflammatory compound in the mussel. And that it works on the rat model. There is also no doubt that it doesn't penetrate the rat gut. I haven't got any evidence that it crosses the human gut — yet. There is no point in trying to experiment with the crude mussel extract on humans. We've got to get the pure stuff and test it."

Gregory travelled to London in 1982 and was interviewed about the mussel extract. He said no more than he told me: that it does contain an anti-inflammatory compound; that in experiments it had reduced rat footpad swelling by half. Present anti-inflammatory drugs only treated the symptoms; the search had to go on for a true anti-arthritic drug that cured the condition that caused it.

He said to the *Yorkshire Post:* "The discovery (at RMIT) is extremely important as a positive step forward towards this goal. If in fact the active ingredient is effective as an anti-arthritic agent, then it will alleviate the suffering of millions."

Gregory is critical of the company's public relations approach. "I believe they are doing themselves harm in the longterm by persisting with PR. I believe there is a compound here that could ultimately do some good. But if they don't watch it they are going to stuff it, and they'll be off the market forever and it's going to be lost.

"On the other side of the coin, Jim Broadbent points out that if it wasn't for these sales in health food shops and chemists, there would be no money and I wouldn't be doing my research work now.

"He walks a tight-rope and he appreciates it; and I appreciate it I suppose. I just hope we get somewhere before some disaster occurs."

* * *

Finally, a medical view...

A leading rheumatologist talked to me about several aspects of arthritis and claimed 'cures'.

Gastro-protection. If the mussel did indeed offer gastro-protection, how important would this be, I asked him? "Any substance," he said, "which can protect the gastric mucosa against the damaging effects of anti-inflammatories is of great interest to rheumatologists and worthy of further investigation. This is a major obstacle to making life bearable for many sufferers from rheumatic disorders. It is one reason why we need a spectrum of anti-inflammatories. Some people react unfavourably in terms of gastric irritation or ulceration to one preparation, but not to another. Very often the hands of the rheumatologist are tied in this respect because there are severe limitations placed on marketing of anti-inflammatories in Australia which are available overseas. These preparations vary, not only in their effect on the gastric mucosa, but also in their efficacy in different individuals."

On *research.* "Research into rheumatic disorders is very much an 'Orphan Annie' in the medical field, and Australia does not spend enough money on medical research as opposed to other forms of research. If an individual or a company has a substance which they feel has potential, there are various avenues open to establishing the effectiveness and safety — or otherwise — of the preparation.

"The first step is to prepare a protocol for a properly controlled study and to agree that the results will be made available whatever the outcome. This may start with a pilot study and then go on to a more fully-fledged study which could be multi-centred or simply be a smaller study repeated in different centres independently. The protocol should be decided with the advice of experts in the field of designing trials in the rheumatic disorders. This is a very expensive business and the possible avenues for obtaining finances are:

1. *The National Health and Medical Research Council.* This body has limited funds and has not been shown to be particularly generous in the field of rheumatic disorders. It sets very high standards for any projects submitted to it for consideration

of subsidy.

2. *Pharmaceutical companies.* They do have resources and if there were a potentially marketable preparation they would be very interested in looking into financing appropriate studies. Of course they would expect "a piece of the action" in due course, but it should be possible to make a mutually suitable arrangement. Again, they would have to be satisfied that the claims had some sort of merit.

3. *Arthritis Foundation.* The Arthritis Foundations in Australia have limited resources, but if the claim has sufficient merit they would certainly be very interested in giving support to raising finances for further research. Again, critical appraisal of the evidence suggested would be essential. I believe the whole thing boils down to a hard critical appraisal of the original evidence and a painstaking piecing together of evidence in increasing volume until, if possible, a clear-cut picture emerges as to the efficacy or otherwise of the substance."

THE END.